Finding Inner Safety

The key to healing, thriving, and overcoming burnout

Dr. Nerina Ramlakhan

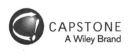

CAPSTONE
A Wiley Brand

Registered office
John Wiley & Sons, Inc., 111 River Street, Hoboken, NJ 07030, USA
John Wiley & Sons Ltd, The Atrium, Southern Gate, Chichester, West Sussex, PO19 8SQ, United Kingdom

Editorial Office
John Wiley & Sons Ltd, The Atrium, Southern Gate, Chichester, West Sussex, PO19 8SQ, United Kingdom

For details of our global editorial offices, customer services, and more information about Wiley products visit us at www.wiley.com.

Wiley also publishes its books in a variety of electronic formats and by print-on-demand. Some content that appears in standard print versions of this book may not be available in other formats.

Library of Congress Cataloging-in-Publication Data is Available:
ISBN 9780857089236 (paperback)
ISBN 9780857089243 (ePub)
ISBN 9780857089250 (ePDF)

Cover Design: Wiley
Cover Image: © Elina Li/Shutterstock

SKY16DE60DF-CDC1-4834-8614-D79C4E0E6E98_033122

For both Nirvanas, past and present

Contents

Contents

Contents

Contents

Message from the Author

When I began writing this book, I soon realized that *all* of me wanted to be wholeheartedly involved – the scientist, the practitioner, the philosopher, the survivor, and the thriver. So, what unfolded, and what you will come across in the four sections of my book, is a blend of the various ingredients that have, over the years, become my USP – I call them my 5Ps. In the blending of these 5Ps, I aim to present to you a more holistic viewpoint, and one that will not only ignite your intellect but also open your heart, nourish your soul, and spur you to action!

Physiology and Psychology

I started out as a scientist. I have a degree in physiology and a doctorate in neurophysiology. And I have also studied psychology and psychiatry. It wasn't long after my postdoctoral work and a couple of short-lived academic posts that I realized I wasn't really interested in being an academic. Actually, I thought I wasn't cut out for the world of work at all until I experienced the 'click' of working in the 'human laboratory' and realized that my real fascination lay in the workings of the mind, body, and spirit. Particularly fascinating were seemingly 'esoteric' concepts and how they might be explained by scientific theory, an interest I could never have pursued if I had stayed in academia, constrained by strict scientific protocols and peer review pressure. I needed to let my mind roam free! Free to find the answers to the Why's that petri dishes and test tubes were never going to give me. I believe this stood me in good stead when I began consulting in corporate environments where many of my clients tended to be more left brain – logical, rational, 'if you can't see it, it doesn't exist' human beings. For such clients, blending esoteric with scientific theories was probably more credible. Perhaps it felt safer too.

Professional Experience

Observations from the 'human laboratory' started back in the 1990s when I headed to London's Square Mile to work in a health-screening clinic. Still wearing a lab coat but this time measuring the health of corporate employees. Since then, I've been measuring people's health, talking to them about their health, observing how life impacts on our health. And not only corporate executives such as law, accountancy, or insurance firms and investment banks. I've also worked with police officers, schoolchildren, lorry drivers driving oil tankers through the night, women recovering from cancer, stressed-out mothers, chief executives and their chauffeurs, famous actors, members of royal families from far-flung exotic places, members of Parliament. And I spent more than a decade working in a psychiatric clinic, The Capio Nightingale Clinic, where, ironically, years before, I'd stayed for a month as an in-patient. Here, I worked with people who had burnt out, people with addictions, people who couldn't sleep, felt depressed, anxious, afraid, and who'd lost hope. In this book I will share snippets of the stories of some of the people I've been privileged to help over the years, showing you how they found inner safety.

Philosophy

When I began my healing journey in 1999, the ancient sciences and philosophies started calling me. Maybe they'd whispered to me first and then I embarked on the journey without realizing I was being guided, woken up. By then I had my degrees, my left brain had been trained and honed by years of academic study and research but the Why's were clamouring for my attention and I needed to look beyond the reductionism of academic research to find more answers. My intuition was telling me that there was so much more to learn. I was feeling things, intuiting things, but unable to understand or trust what I was feeling. As Einstein said: 'The intuitive mind is a sacred gift and the rational mind is a faithful servant.'

So, I returned to my lineage of Hinduism, took a foray into Buddhism, explored the ancient sciences of Ayurveda and traditional Chinese medicine and found more answers.

Always Practical

I have learnt so much over the years and amassed so many tools and resources. I always share these in my work as well as practising them myself. I share nothing that I don't practise myself – *physician heal thyself*. Many of the tools I'll share with you might seem like small things – how could they possibly make a difference? But there are times when we are tired, burnt out, and feeling at a loss and we don't have the energy to make big changes. I have found that these small changes are a good starting point and might even be the tipping point that can help to lever you out if you are stuck in a rut.

Personal Insight

Throughout *Finding Inner Safety* I invite you to think about yourself and how my words relate to you. The issue of feeling safe is a deeply personal one. How could I not ask you to consider your own thoughts, feelings, and experiences?

I also share elements of my own story . . . I have hinted at this in my previous books but this time I felt it was necessary to share more. This book is definitely not a memoir but I share because I want you to know that I have lived what I talk about, and not just studied it or worked with it. It is amongst my most important values to 'be the change', which means that what I offer you comes from deep within me. I am someone who has lived and continues to live deeply and, for some reason, has been given a voice of influence and countless opportunities to help others through my own experience.

Ironically, writing *Finding Inner Safety* took me on a deep journey of healing in which I realized that not only did I need to stop downplaying my own story, but I had something to share that could help others. I found a deep compassion – for myself and for my family and ancestors and the struggles they'd undergone. And I explored one of my most important Why's? Why am I here? According to Hindu and Buddhist philosophy, we are here for a reason, to fulfil a life purpose – this is called our *dharma*. I have long realized that in doing the work that I do I am fulfilling my *dharma* but I hadn't realized how much writing this book was a vital part of that life purpose. As I wrote, something settled in me and I found an even deeper sense of inner safety. This is what happens when we find our *dharma* and I have watched this happen with many others too.

Many of you will have your own incredible stories too and in all of these stories, including mine, there are common themes – uprootings, awakenings, and realizations; dealing with challenges, going into one's depths to source clarity and resources, finding mentors and building supports that enable you to emerge differently with a deeper sense of inner safety.

I trust that you find inspiration, hope, and energy to embark on your journey. Maybe the sharing of my story will help you to understand your own story, shed your own tears, and find your own liberation.

My book is organized into four main parts, together with a Prologue, Introduction, and Epilogue. I start by telling a personal story that showed me, without doubt, why safety matters and where it really comes from.

Part One: The Illusion of Safety

As I write this book, we are in the midst of a pandemic unlike anything any of us have ever been through. But even before this we had been living as compromised human beings, stress levels rising, mental health issues common, and, especially amongst our young, people are unable to sleep. But I believe that these aren't the real epidemics; at the heart of it we have become so disconnected from our true selves – our souls – and lost the ability to feel safe. In our technology-driven world we've also lost connection with others; for many people relating has become virtual, superficial, text-character-based. Man is, after all, a social animal, and it is in the building of authentic and deep connections that real safety can also be found.

What are we talking about when we talk about feeling safe? I propose that there are four levels at which we might seek to feel safe – physical, emotional, mental, and spiritual. Human beings are complex and we feel safest when we are integrated and whole on these four levels – physical, emotional, mental, and spiritual. I will invite you to think about how you feel on each of these levels. Thus, you can become more intimately acquainted with your unique relationship with feeling safe and, importantly, discover where the healing lies for you.

Part Two: When the Nervous System Is Nervous

In the second part, I introduce you to the physiology of feeling safe, the nervous system and the vital role it plays in helping us to survive or thrive. I believe that understanding the workings of your nervous system is crucial to your being able to navigate safely in a world that often feels unsafe. I also describe an important and relatively new physiological theory that I myself stumbled upon only a few years ago while working on this book and a particularly painful stage of my own healing journey. Today, this theory and its practical application is becoming increasingly important in the understanding and treatment of trauma both at the clinical level and in everyday life.

Part Three: Nature Cures

This part of the book is very dear to me. Initially, the scientist in me worried that what I was writing was whimsical and fluffy and that I'd be called a tree hugger! In order to write it, I needed to retreat into myself for a while. It was August 2021 and in London we hoped we'd come out of the pandemic. People weren't sure what to do with themselves; it felt as if the world was in a lull – a perfect time to be still and write about safety from a different perspective and one that even my 'gurus', neuroscientist Dr Stephen Porges and trauma therapist Deb Dana, hadn't written about – the healing potential of trees and their ability to show us how to feel safe. These respected professionals are considered by many to be amongst the top pioneers in the relatively new field of 'safety science'.

My gut or intuition was guiding me strongly here, driven by the question: What is the counterbalance to all of noise out there? The opinions and divisiveness in our world? The uncertainty that we're all facing at the moment? All of this serves to take us even further away from feelings of safety and surety. Can trees, just by virtue of how they exist and operate, demonstrate to us all what feeling safe really means? In this section of my book I show you that they truly can.

My aim in writing this book is to take you deep. We can't 'do' feeling safe unless we are prepared to plunge our depths. This means going back to the source or the roots of our relationship with feeling safe, where we came from, through tramlines of parental and ancestral DNA from our parents and back to their parents, and their parents too. And even beyond . . . I started thinking – what if we go back to our very beginnings on earth? Can we learn something meaningful about how to feel safe in our changing world? According to James Lovelock, the prize-winning creator of the *Gaia* hypothesis, we are inextricably connected to our planet, to Mother Earth and nature.

In this third part, I write about the unexpected muse who turned up at the right time and helped me to deepen my understanding of the roots of our safety. Here I write about our relationship with nature – and trees in particular – what they can teach us about feeling safe and their amazing capacity to heal. I believe it can also teach us how to break free from patterns of survival and truly thrive. For too long we have been obsessed with our world of technology, speed, and consumerism and this is what we have looked to in order to feel secure. Right now, with our whole world in chaos and crisis, we need a different perspective and one that brings us back to who we are, our true nature.

Part Four: Doing the Real Work (of Finding Inner Safety)

The final part of my book is practical. Here, I share the resources that I have been learning about, practising myself, and teaching thousands of people for years. These are the practices – some of them very simple – that I have been sharing with people for decades, as well as practising myself.

In this resources section I share the tools that are based on my unique methodology. I take you through a process that is focused on bringing safety to those four crucial levels – physical, emotional, mental, and spiritual – that I describe in Part One. Ideally, you will work your way through the practices and decide which ones work best for you. The nature of this work is deeply personal after all. However, I recommend that you start with the RESET practice, as my experience has shown me that preparing the foundations in this way sets you up to do the deeper work that comes later. I hesitated to call this section a 'toolbox' but I suppose it could be considered to be that, as embarking on the journey of building inner safety really is about 'Doing the Work', a label which I use throughout my book and which I ask you to become familiar with too. This is about doing the 'the Work' of becoming a more evolved human being, more self-actualized. I will share with you an array of tools that I've learnt from others, developed and practised myself, and shared with countless others. Over time, you will become more adept at selecting the tools you need at different stages of doing your own work.

In conclusion, *Finding Inner Safety* ends on a message of hope and joy. I am writing this book at a time when many feel hopeless, afraid, and even suspicious. All around us there is chaotic, uncomfortable change and we don't know where it is taking us.

However, it is time – at least for the sake of our younger generation, the future of our species – to spread a new type of contagion. One of realistic optimism and joy even in the face of life's inevitable suffering. I say 'realistic' because this isn't about toxic, fake positivity. This is about finding those moments of real hope, real joy, real gratitude, and real kinship that do exist . . . and spreading it. We're all connected and we're all in this together. We might feel we have no influence but we all do. Each one of us has the power to tap into something deep within us – a wellspring of safety from which true thriving is created.

Acknowledgements

Writing a book is a solitary experience and doing this while the whole world was in the throes of the Covid-19 pandemic and we were all in lockdown could have been a lonely experience had it not been for the friends and angels who anchored me, held me safe, and came along on the journey.

I have many to thank . . .

Not least Mira – my canine soulmate from the streets of Cyprus who arrived, uncannily, just at the right time. We soothed each other's nervous systems and made each other feel safe. I'm not sure who was rescuing whom. You are a joy in my life!

Beautiful friendships were made thanks to the River Thames, just at my doorstep. Thank you, my river buddies, Denise Yeats, Jessie Laute, Luisa Kuramapu, Amaresh, Rick, and Jam Cam, crazy human beings who help me to laugh and breathe deeply – the only way to self-regulate when immersing in icy waters. Strangely, the murky but steady waters of the river provided the most magical support for writing this book, especially when I was stuck for words or just plain stuck in my head.

Soul sisters and dear friendships that have deepened even throughout the isolation of the last year – Gosia Gorna, Carolyn Kolasinski, Lindsay Doy, Kirsten Samuel, Heena Thaker, and more recently the divinely special Jackie Boothe. Thank you for listening to me, and for holding space when tears flowed in the unveiling process. Your voice messages were such a welcome relief from the voice in my own head during those isolation months.

Yasmin Ibrahim for being there just at the right time and the amazing connections that have resulted from you turning up on that fateful day. Heartfelt thanks to you and the Bingham Riverhouse for helping me get my mojo back and remember that the best form of healing takes place when you're shaking it out on the dance floor.

To my wonderful support team at the Adia PR agency – notably Laura Coppock and Ruth Shearman and my lovely VA Polly Buckley. You all bent over backwards to help me protect precious writing time. Kerry-Lyn Stanton-Downes who has held space and walked with me since the inception of this book.

Deepest gratitude for my ancestors whose presence and guidance I felt throughout, not least in my dreams. Funny how the dreams have stopped since submitting the manuscript. I have written this book to honour your journey, your tenacity and courage, attributes which I feel ingrained in my deepest taproots.

For the family that I chose in this lifetime and especially Mum – I can't wait to see you again. It has been too long. Dad, you always said I should be a writer and you were right. I miss you.

To my wonderful friend, agent, and Book Angel Wendy Yorke for your unwavering support and belief in me and this book throughout the whole process. I am so grateful to you.

And finally, thank you to my daughter, Maya Nirvana, my best teacher. You continue to both inspire and test me and I love you.

Prologue:
Lost and Found

It is 5 o'clock in the afternoon and the sun beats down on the Portuguese mountains and my bare shoulders. My throat is dry and sore, parched from thirst and my futile screams for help. A few minutes ago, I turned my right ankle sharply when I scrambled down the slope, searching in vain for the trail I'd started out on two hours ago. The pain is irrelevant at this point. What started out as a 30-minute run in the Portuguese mountains that I've done many times before has gone horribly wrong and I'm lost lost lost . . .

I'm aware that my breathing is jagged and panicky, and I force myself to exhale slowly, trying in vain to take control of my body. Cursing myself for not having told anyone back at the yoga retreat that I was going for a run. No one saw me leave. I have no phone, no torch. Just me in my running kit with a watch. Dinner is at 7 p.m. Will anyone notice I'm not there? Will my friend raise the alarm? Will they send a search party for me? Can I sleep out here in the mountains? What about wild animals? Will I survive? What will happen to my daughter? Will I ever see her again? Panic mounts and I give up the battle to deepen my breath.

An hour later the sun dips down behind the mountains. Nature is oblivious to my terror and a golden-red glow spreads across the sky. I see butterflies of every colour flirting with flowers, a herd of wild boar gaze at me with disinterest, a leggy fawn spots me and darts into the undergrowth. I'm a nature girl but I'm in no mood to appreciate. Right now, I'd give anything to be on a packed commuter train in the middle of a concrete jungle. Thirst leads me down to the depths of the valley and, fighting my way through wild grasses and thorny bushes, I lie on my belly and drink gratefully from a gushing spring. The sky darkens and night falls. I've never felt so lonely. In desperation I bargain and pray – dear God please help me. Show me the way back. I promise I'll be a better mother, daughter, sister, friend, human being . . . No response.

Night time falls and I'm walking, stumbling along by the light of the stars and moon sliver. I abandon an attempt to shelter in a deserted barn. What *is* that rustling noise? Are those snakes or rats I hear? I had thought I could stay here until sunrise when I might have a better view of the valley but I can't do it; I have to keep moving. By now I'm freezing and I fashion a makeshift cloak from a torn plastic bag lying amongst the rubble in the barn.

As the light levels drops, strangely, so does my panic. I have less choice now as I can hardly even see my feet.

At times I have no idea whether I'm still on the trail but all I can do is keep going. As I walk, something approaching a sense of calm settles over me. Maybe I'm too exhausted to be afraid – by now I've been on my feet for more than five hours. It's not that I've given up but that somehow the voice in my head has changed. It's become quieter and steadier. It tells me to keep walking, just keep putting one foot in front of the other. My focus seems to have shifted from looking out there and trying to find the way to 'in here'. . . I seem to be tuning in to an inner satellite navigation system that I didn't even know I had. As I do so, a **deep sense of safety** spreads through my body and I know without a doubt that I'm going to be absolutely fine. An hour later and I find myself on a wide road that takes me back to the retreat. I've found my way home.

Over to You . . .

Dear Reader, have you ever been so lost, so stuck in a situation that you've wondered how you might leave it or even survive? You've felt overwhelmed, fearful, sick with worry. But somehow you came through it? Or maybe you haven't. Maybe you're in there right now, feeling afraid and alone.

I know this feeling only too well as I've felt unsafe and lost so many times in my life. Until I learned how to find my way back. What happened to me in the mountains was terrifying – sure I screamed and hollered, panicked and bargained – but I found within me a deep state of trust and inner safety. At some point, I knew I'd find my way back and this happened even before I'd arrived back at the retreat . . .

It hasn't always been this way. I've travelled a magical journey and learnt a great deal. I've learnt how to find safety even in the messiest and most traumatic of circumstances. Throughout grief, loss, and devastation . . . I've learnt how to find deep safety within myself and then move from this place of trust and inner knowing. I eventually found this place when I was lost in the mountains and, from this inner compass, I found my way back home.

At the heart of it, this is what I talk about when I talk about feeling safe. It is about finding within a place of profound inner stillness from which you can deal with whatever turmoil is around you. It is an inner place from which you relate to life especially when it is tough, confusing, heart-breaking.

We need this in today's world which has become so fast-paced and chaotic. Sometimes there's so much sensory input coming at us and we just don't know which way to turn – all around us are clamouring voices saying 'This way! That way!'

How do we discern in such uncertainty? How do we choose from a place of grounded steadiness and calm? Not from a place of adrenalized fear and panic? We find within us a place of inner safety – it's in all of us, not just me. It really does reside in all of us and I don't mean this in a fluffy, esoteric way; **each one of us is wired physiologically with access to this place of inner deep knowing and safety.** Many people go through their lives never finding it but I'm going to show you how to find it in this book.

The thing about feeling safe is that when we've found it, truly found it, we can respond to life differently. We can take risks, open our hearts to love, leave toxic relationships, stop doing work that is burning us out day after day. We can truly thrive.

What I have learnt is amazing but at the same time so simple and I have been privileged to be able to share these learnings or 'tools' in my books, workshops, on stage, TV, and radio for over 20 years and in a way that has made a profound difference for thousands of people.

I am looking forward to sharing with you too.

Nerina Ramlakhan, May 2021

Introduction: Why Feeling Safe Matters

To feel safe is one of our greatest and most primal drives.

We come into this life on an ongoing quest to find inner safety from the moment of birth until the moment of death. When a baby is born it leaves the warm, dark, safe cocoon of its mother's womb and arrives into a harsh, bright, noisy environment which probably feels profoundly unsafe. In those first moments after the birth, in both mother and child, levels of oxytocin (the love and trust-building hormone) and endorphins are at peak levels to maximize bonding between the baby and mother. To enable the baby to feel safe. Skin-to-skin contact between mother and child deepens the feeling of safety. Once the baby has an embodied experience of safety, it moves to suckle and breastfeed and an even deeper connection between mother and child is formed.

Feeling safe is essential to our ability to both survive and thrive. As Deb Dana, leading trauma therapist says, 'With our first breath, we embark on a lifelong quest to feel safe in our bodies, in our environments, and in our relationship with others.'

But why is a 'sleep expert' writing about feeling safe?

I started writing this book 15 years ago and ended up writing three books on sleep in the meantime. The world needed books on sleep; technology had well and truly landed on the scene, the speed of life ramped up, and we struggled to slow down . . . and sleep. Globally, the sleep industry is now worth billions of pounds with our state-of-the-art mattresses, pillows, blackout blinds, aromatherapy candles, meditation apps . . . We've come a long way since the hunter-gatherer lying on a mat of leaves in a cave.

I never set out to be a sleep expert. I discovered a knack for helping people to sleep (largely driven by my own long-standing issues with insomnia), wrote my first book *Tired but Wired* and boom! Now, I'm called a sleep expert.

'We sleep when we feel safe' was what I started saying in presentations and people took notice. They wrote this sentence down.

I knew that the real key to helping people to sleep was to help them to feel safe.

And I knew the key to helping people to thrive was to help them to feel safe.

Our nervous system is designed along the premise of:

Is the world safe or unsafe?

We're constantly, subconsciously, scanning our environment, relating to the world around us. Our nervous system judges whether we're safe or unsafe, whether we're free to thrive or we need to fight to survive.

This neurophysiological judgement – safe or unsafe? – affects everything. The way we live and relate to others. The way our bodies behave – our health and wellbeing. The choices we make.

Is it safe to cross the road now?
Is it safe to leave this job?
Is it safe to stay in this relationship?

And more recently, with the Covid-19 pandemic:

Is it safe to hug this person?
Is it safe for me to leave my house?
Is it safe for me to have this vaccine/not have this vaccine?

The Covid-19 pandemic has well and truly placed the issue of feeling safe on the agenda. But in reality, it has been there for a while; for too long, people have been walking around in survival mode – I've been observing and measuring this for the last 20-odd years. The speed of life ramping up, becoming so chaotic that our nervous systems have collectively, subconsciously habituated to survival, to feeling unsafe.

In other words, we've got used to *living in the wrong part of our nervous system*. We've got used to feeling on edge, over-stimulated, unable to stop, afraid to stop, sick when we stop. We're constantly running away from hidden threat. We don't feel safe and we don't even realize that.

I began to see and measure this decade ago and the desire to write this book began to take form. But then I didn't have all of my answers. And, at the end of the day, it's all about timing. At the time, publishers didn't want it – they thought no one would understand or want to buy a book about feeling safe. Or at least, the ordinary man on the street might not want to buy a book on feeling safe, but in another world, the scientific and trauma therapy community, interest in 'safety science' was slowly gaining momentum. When I came across the work of Stephen Porges and read his book *The Polyvagal Theory*, several pennies dropped, and my own life changed. Something settled in me, maybe my own nervous system settled as I discovered missing links. I fell in love with Stephen Porges' work, but his book might not be accessible to all.

From a Polyvagal perspective, a focus on autonomic balance obfuscates the importance of the phylogenetically-ordered response hierarchy of how the autonomic nervous system reacts to challenges.

This book, I hoped and prayed, was just that so I finally settled down to write *Finding Inner Safety*.

But the world still wasn't quite ready.

In February 2020, I sat with the commissioning editor for one of the biggest publishing houses in the world talking about this book. 'It'll be a hard sell for our sales team. People won't know what "feeling safe" means', she said.

Three weeks later we hit the pandemic. Suddenly, everyone is not feeling safe. Everyone is rushing out bulk-buying toilet paper, rice, and pasta, and wearing masks. The urban hunter-gatherer was well and truly in survival mode.

It is time to reset the nervous system if we're going to thrive.

A Personal Agenda

Life keeps giving me opportunities to talk to people about feeling safe. Recently, in the magical setting of Ashridge Business School in the UK, I spoke to an international group of leaders about the nervous system and feeling safe. One of them, a successful businessman who leads a large international team in a well-known accountancy firm, came up to me afterwards and said that he hadn't realized that what he'd been feeling for years was 'unsafe' and that my words had been a 'wake-up' for him.

As I mentioned right at the beginning when I shared my 'ingredients', my work comes not only from the head but also from my heart and soul. Feeling safe matters to me. Maybe because for more than half of my life I haven't felt safe.

When you've grown up feeling fear every day of your life, the sensation of fear becomes normal. You habituate to it. In fact, it wasn't until I was 31 years old and a therapist in the psychiatric unit I'd just been admitted to asked me 'How are you feeling?' that I realized that I'd been afraid most of my life – not excited (what I'd told myself).

What was I afraid of? At the time I didn't know. All I know is that there was a bad feeling stuck in my body and I perpetually felt unsafe. Often it served me well – it drove me to run fast and I did – completing seven marathons and over 40 triathlons. Feeling unsafe drove me to achieve, to get stuff done, to win, to be the best. But I was afraid most of the time. My moods oscillated between high energy, verging on hyperactive, in which I was the life and soul of the party and then withdrawn, depressed, and exhausted – very few people saw me in this state but I was known for cancelling social engagements at short notice. Both states derive from living in the wrong part of the nervous system, from running on fear.

According to Elisabeth Kübler-Ross, psychiatrist and pioneer in near-death studies who introduced the Kübler-Ross model of the five stages of grief:

There are only two emotions: love and fear. All positive emotions come from love, all negative emotions from fear. From love flows happiness, contentment, peace and joy. From fear comes anger, hate, anxiety, and guilt. It's true that there are only two primary emotions, love and fear. But it's more accurate to say that there is only love or fear, for we cannot feel these two emotions together, at exactly the same time. They are opposites. If we're in fear, we are not in a place of love. When we are in a place of love, we cannot be in a place of fear.

When we feel unsafe, everything comes from FEAR. When we feel safe, everything stems from LOVE. So, we're either running away from life or running towards it. What are you doing? Do you know?

At the point of my 'breakdown' (for simplicity's sake, I'm going to call it that for now) I was running away from life not towards it. And fast.

There are several reasons why, up to this point, I was programmed to run on fear, for example, I have a high ACE (Adverse Childhood Experiences) score. Throughout my childhood I witnessed and experienced first-hand my father's rages. I watched and heard him beat my mother – sometimes in front of us, sometimes behind closed doors.

After one beating, my mother was forced to flee with my brother, leaving my sister and me at home with my dad.

I was 10 years old and didn't know if I'd ever see my mother or brother again. For days we tiptoed around my father and then one day he went out in the car and, after a few hours, returned with them. No one spoke of this event again and I 'forgot' about it. It was decades later – in fact, while writing this book, that my brother reminded me of this incident. This was one of several significant turning points for me. One that enabled me to join several dots and understand why, for more than half of my life, I'd made the choices I'd made, including the following:

My first suicide attempt was when I was 17 years old. I attempted suicide another two times before my mid-30s.

I suffered from eating disorders until the age of 34.

I have been arrested for shoplifting. Charges were dropped when kind police officers realized I was mentally unstable. Weeks later I had a breakdown. I was 31 and spent a month in a psychiatric clinic where, years later, I was headhunted to work for more than a decade.

My beloved sister who had, for most of my childhood, been my primary caregiver, died suddenly and traumatically in 2002.

Two marriages ended. The second one suddenly and traumatically.

In the past, I have been diagnosed with bipolar disorder and complex post-traumatic stress disorder.

I no longer consider myself to have these or any other psychiatric labels nor to be a victim of my life.

I share my story not so that you can say 'poor Nerina'. It is among my highest values to be authentic, real, and honest. I want you to know that *I* know how it feels to feel so profoundly unsafe that I don't want to go on anymore. When we hit rock bottom, one of the most common feelings is feeling so alone, as if no one else could possibly understand. Often this is also tinged with shame and guilt – 'I shouldn't be feeling like this'. Or even 'Have I brought this on myself? Is this what I deserve?'

I want you to know that you are not alone and that I do understand.

I do not consider myself to be a survivor but a thriver. I now run towards life – not away from it. Love sponsors my choices. I no longer want to leave this world, as I once did.

I have found safety in this world, in spite of the world.

Mostly, I share my story in the hope that it might inspire you to keep going and trust that if you are prepared to do the work, something will happen to you – you too will discover a deep inner safety even in the face of adversity – and in spite of the world.

I have written this book for all of you who are feeling as if for too long you've been running in survival mode and feeling afraid. At the time of writing this book, we seem to be emerging from a pandemic that has been traumatic for many. For some people, old wounds have been opened, some of which they inherited and didn't even know they were carrying. For others, the events of the past year in themselves have caused wounding and trauma. I offer you my words in the hope that you can all receive something good from them whether your lived experience is big T or little T. By this I mean, whether you have been through the big traumas of life – the severe life-threatening events – or the small traumas that are more subtle and personal but still affect your health and quality of life. My book is for anyone who wants to know what it means to feel safe. It is for anyone who truly wants to thrive.

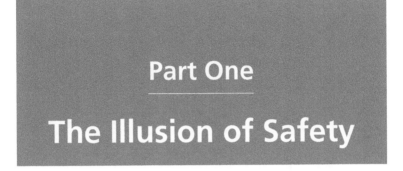

Part One

The Illusion of Safety

Habituation to Survival

1
What Does Feeling Safe Mean?

'If you want to improve the world, start by making people feel safer.'

—Stephen Porges

Stuck in Unhelpful Patterns

Over the years, people have come to me because they can't sleep, they are exhausted and have no energy, they feel anxious, restless, or they're just plain unhappy. Sometimes they've been signed off work – they've had a breakdown or burnt out. I met many people like this when I worked at the psychiatric clinic for 10 years.

Whatever it is that's brought them to me, they've got to a point where things are just not working for them anymore. Occasionally, they want something different, often they don't know that something different is possible.

Usually, they'd been stuck on a treadmill, caught up in patterns of behaviour and unhelpful cycles that they just couldn't change until they hit a point where they had to stop. Often, they didn't even realize how bad they were feeling. Many years ago, I worked with a senior trader and his team of 80 traders in a Japanese investment bank. He'd given me a 20-minute slot at 7 a.m. in one of their team meetings to speak to his team about stress. Perhaps a crazy gig but back then, at the start of my speaking career, I was pretty much saying 'yes' to everything. I said yes to this piece of work, not really realizing how challenging it would be. We were in a large boardroom around a long oval table, and I was at one end of the table. Even at 7 a.m., they were a noisy bunch and the energy in the room felt discordant and a bit chaotic. Fifty traders eating breakfast and fuelling up on energy drinks and caffeine for the work that lay ahead of them. Young, bright, and sparky, they didn't really want to listen to me talking about burnout. I gave them all a stress questionnaire to complete and they laughingly boasted about their scores. The head trader proudly shared his score, the highest in the room, of 85 (the scores shouldn't be higher than 35). He said to me 'I feel fine'. He looked like death, his skin covered in eczema and very overweight. I came away from the session feeling deflated. I found out a month later that he'd had a breakdown and was in a psychiatric clinic.

Sometimes we choose to ignore the symptoms. It doesn't feel safe to acknowledge them. We just keep going until we can't anymore. I know I used to do this and usually I'd get sick as soon as I stopped. Does this ring bells with you too?

This is no longer my pattern, and I am able to work with so many people who are ready to do things in a different way. We work with each other. I show them some ways out of these patterns – resets if you like – and things start to change. The changes take place within them and outside of them. Most of them can't go back to their old patterns but sometimes a few do. They can't find the resources/willpower/energy/reasons to do it differently and end up eventually in a version of the same place.

But many do shift and change.

They find their voice, speak up, refusing to do life in that way anymore.

They leave the relationship or challenge the status quo.

They leave the job.

They move house or state or country.

They ask for help.

This is finding safety.

When You Don't Know if You Feel Safe or Not

The thing about safety is that we might not even realize that we have it or that we don't have it.

The way I see it is that there are four options:

1. Consciously safe – I feel safe and I'm aware of this.
2. Unconsciously safe – I feel safe but I don't realize this. All is well in my world and I'm not giving it too much thought.
3. Consciously unsafe – I don't feel safe. This doesn't feel good.
4. Unconsciously unsafe – not feeling safe and not even realizing it. Numbed out. Habituated to survival.

It's confusing, isn't it? Do you have an idea where you might be in this mix? And we can feel a combination of the four different states at any given time.

The body is wise – it wants to keep us safe for our survival. Sometimes this means not being able to feel because whatever we've experienced is simply too big, it would overwhelm us. So, we learn to shut down, numb out, freeze the feelings out. I will tell you more about this in the next chapter when we look at the workings of the nervous system and how it protects us from threat.

But first, let me ask you, how are you feeling right now? Are you feeling safe or unsafe?

The process of growing, healing, learning, and evolving is moving through states of safety in an ever-deepening spiral (Figure 1.1) in which we move from unconsciously unsafe (not knowing) to consciously unsafe (an uncomfortable awareness, discomfort with life) to unconsciously safe (feeling good and not even realizing it) to consciously safe (I am safe and I know it!). We become more adept at spotting our patterns, our symptoms, the energy states that give us more information about where we are on this spiral. This knowing can be so reassuring; we don't have to move to medicate or pathologize it. We simply know that we're going through another stage of our persona growth and evolution, and we get better with sitting in the discomfort of it and resourcing ourselves with the right tools. And I'm here to help you with this!

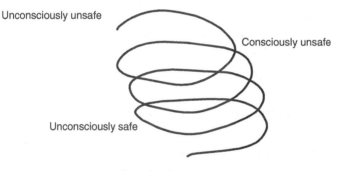

Figure 1.1 The spiral journey of finding inner safety.

Unconsciously Unsafe

Here we have no self-awareness. We don't realize that what we are feeling is unsafe because we haven't allowed ourselves to pause. Maybe life hasn't made us stop and feel. This is a sort of blissful ignorance.

We might numb out with:

- Food
- Catch-up TV and Netflix
- Work
- Sex
- Prescription medication
- Exercise
- Alcohol
- Drugs
- Obsessive busyness
- Work (even if we hate what we're doing)
- Social media
- Obsessive control over our environment
- Perfectionism
- Self-harming.

We might also 'numb' out with excessive preoccupation with how we are or aren't sleeping. This is often what brings people to my door. They can't

- get to sleep;
- stay asleep;
- get enough sleep;
- stop waking up at night;
- stop grinding their teeth;
- stop the thoughts at night; and
- stop crying out in their sleep.

Because they don't feel safe. (And don't forget, we sleep when we feel safe.)

When we're unconsciously unsafe we stay stuck in unhappy situations – at work, at home, in our relationships. We don't speak out. We hold ourselves tight. We grind our teeth. We live in hypervigilance without even realizing that we're constantly on the lookout for threat. We keep trying to overcome without realizing that what is driving us is the constant background noise of fear and anxiety.

Often people habituate to a level of unhappiness (and un-safety) and they stop questioning it, noticing it – as I described previously with the banker and his team.

It's odd but there's a level of 'safety' in numbed out habituation – do you agree?

Consciously Unsafe

Now we know what we're dealing with.

Maybe we've been brought to this point by burning out, breaking down, or breaking through. Whatever the route that brought us this point, we've arrived in a place of knowing this isn't good. This is not how I want to live my life. Something needs to change. I want something different.

Now you start to feel. Really feel. Your nervous system is lit up and activated. Your nervous system is nervous. You might feel dissatisfied, angry, grief-stricken, afraid, heartbroken, lost, confused, desperate. There are times when you might even feel hopeless, exhausted, and depressed. What's the point?

It's normal to start feeling when we reach this point of realization. This is the thawing out of numbed out, long-frozen feelings. If we allow this process, sit with it, breathe through it, there will be the proverbial light at the end of the tunnel . . . I'm going to show you how to do this.

Unconsciously Safe

This is a strange one. How could we be feeling safe but not knowing that we are? We might have become so caught up in feeling 'not safe' that we have again habituated to the 'symptoms' of this stage. Until life starts to give us these moments.

I call them 'glimmers and glimpses'. Moments when we find ourselves laughing at something. An unexpected bubbling up of mirth from the depths of our being. We surprise ourselves at the sound of our voice because we haven't genuinely laughed for so long.

Feelings of contentment and peace – sometimes for no particular reason other than just feeling good in our own skin, as the French say 'Bien dans sa peau'.

And it may well be that nothing has particularly changed 'out there' but we've found something deep within ourselves, something 'in here'. Something strong and anchoring. We know we'll be OK no matter what happens in our external world.

The first time I felt this was in 1999. I was sitting on a veranda in Brisbane having left my marriage, my job, suddenly stopped taking prescription mood stabilizing meds (against my doctor's advice). To all intents and purposes, I was free falling, going cold turkey. So, there I was sipping a latte and trying to pour my feelings into my journal in the hope of ridding myself of the uncomfortable feelings of fear and loneliness.

Then – and it felt like it happened in a moment – I looked up from my writing and everything looked different, more vivid. I felt as if I was viewing nature for the first time ever. Suddenly the greens were greener, the birdsong louder, the feeling of spring sunshine on my cool skin somehow more delicious. My senses were alive and dancing. I felt joyful, peaceful, grateful – and for no particular reason that I can identify. Nothing had changed in my external world. It was just a moment. But it was an important moment and one in which something shifted in my internal world that was to change my life forever.

This was my first conscious experience of feeling safe – although I didn't call it that at the time. I just knew that I'd experienced a deep feeling of contentment, peace unlike anything I'd ever felt before and that I wanted more of this. Importantly, I knew I could have more of this – I just needed to keep slowing down and coming back to this place within me.

What exactly happened on that veranda in Brisbane?

Some might call it:

- An awakening
- A moment of grace
- An encounter with God
- A shift in consciousness
- A breakthrough.

In my effort to understand, I have read so many books that have described such moments in religious, spiritual, and even scientific terms. My mind always wants to understand.

What I do know is that that was my first conscious taste of feeling safe. Have you ever felt this too? If so, what was your experience?

Consciously Safe

This is a destination. It is the light at the end of the tunnel.

Feeling safe is a deeply embodied feeling. It resides in the body. I have to keep using these words because I want to move you away from viewing safety as a thought process – I feel safe because I have good friends, I feel safe because my wife loves me, I feel safe because I've been promoted, I feel safe because I have money in the bank.

I'm not denying that these aspects are important but my main goal in writing this book is to help you to find a deeply internalized sense of safety so that even in the absence of these desirables you can feel anchored, grounded, strong, and resourceful (as shown in Figure 1.2).

This is true safety.

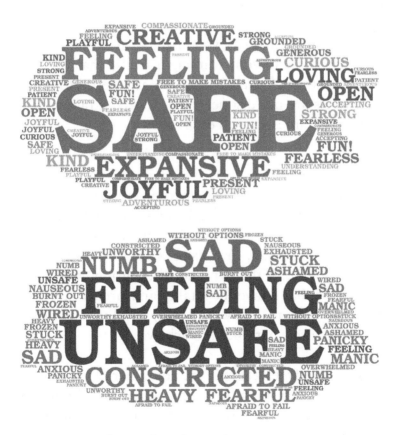

Figure 1.2 Feeling Safe and Unsafe.

Because life is so imperfect, so changeable. We actually have far less control over it than we believe we have.

Four Levels of Safety

Human beings are complex. We are multidimensional beings. As such, safety can reside within us on four different levels.

As I describe these levels, you might wish to think about how they apply to you. You might realize that you feel very safe at some levels but less so at others. However, these levels are not distinct or separate but rather, they connect and interact with each other.

Physical

I am physically safe in my environment, I have a roof over my head, I have enough food and water. I have enough money. My family and I are warm and protected from external threat. In Maslow's Hierarchy of Needs this is the base of the pyramid. Feeling physically safe also means that I have the vitality and strength to fight threat if I have to. I have the energy to live a fulfilling life, to achieve what I need to achieve.

There is also feeling safe in the container of your body, knowing that it is strong, vital, flexible, and adaptable. That it can withstand and endure. That it is resourceful.

As the poet John O'Donohue says, '*The body is your clay home, your only home in the universe.*' When we don't feel safe in our bodies, we might feel weak, powerless, afraid, stuck, or rigid. We lose trust in ourselves. Lack of safety can show up in the body in all sorts of way, including insomnia and restlessness, and even pain. Feeling numb, or ungrounded, is also common when we don't feel safe in our bodies.

Emotional

When I feel safe emotionally, I have connection in my life in the form of warm and loving relationships. I have the emotional flexibility to bounce back from disappointment, frustration, and loss. It is safe for me to feel a range of emotions from anger, sadness, and fear to happiness, playfulness, peace, and joy. It is safe for me to feel whatever I need to feel, whatever I am feeling in this moment. I trust to ask for help and lean on others for support in times of crisis. I trust to allow myself to open up and show others who I am. I trust to open up to loving another even though I could get hurt.

When I don't feel safe emotionally, I shut myself down. I don't trust others and I am wary and judgemental. I isolate myself from others. I am avoidant in relationships, looking for reasons to leave, or I am overly anxious in relationships, constantly seeking approval, reassurance, and validation. I don't trust myself to speak up, so I hold myself back, afraid to show others who I am. I grind my teeth at night because there is so much I want to say but I don't feel safe to. It is not safe to feel so I 'numb out' with exercise, food, sex, drugs, mindless TV, alcohol . . . (feel free to add your own).

Mental

When I feel safe mentally, I know when to say No and when to say Yes. I feel focused and en-missioned. I can tap into my creativity and I trust my intuition. My time is precious, and I know how to use it. In these times of information overload, I know when to stop and rest my mind and I feel safe to do so. I know how to recognize and override any tendencies to pessimism and self-flagellation and I know how to calm these tendencies when they do inevitably arise.

When we feel safe mentally, we are able to create boundaries in how we use our time so we can stay focused without burning ourselves out. We know when to say No and we are not afraid to say it. We are not ruled by the 'mad monkey' in our brain that says we can't stop.

When you don't feel safe on this level you have to stay leaned in, stuck in striving mode. You are ruled by must do's, should do's, have to do's . . . and yet it's never good enough. You hardly notice or celebrate our successes. You play them down or you might even feel ashamed of them. You suffer from imposter syndrome and extreme perfectionism.

Not feeling safe on the mental level can spill into the body in the form of tightness and rigidity; creaking and aching joints; back pain; tightness of jaw, neck, and shoulders; inability to digest food and irritable bowel. You lie in bed unable to sleep, fretting and wired from the day, unable to let go. Holding yourself tight in this way can eventually cause exhaustion, chronic fatigue, and burnout.

Spiritual

This is the ultimate safety level.

I trust the process of life. Even when things are going wrong, I have faith that I will be OK. I am able to connect with something beyond myself and this calms, reassures, and bolsters me. I know what is important to me – what I value – and I am committed to living my life according to these values even if this sometimes causes personal sacrifice. I can rise above the messiness of a situation and see the learning for me, even the gift. I can see the Why.

When we are spiritually safe, we feel a sense of trust. We have faith even in times of adversity. We are aligned with our values and are not afraid to live our lives by them. We continually search for meaning, knowing that it matters. We refuse to play the victim, never giving up on life, recognizing that each wound takes us into deeper healing and greater strength. We courageously seek to understand our unique purpose in life – our *dharma* – knowing that this brings us ultimate joy and deepest safety.

What Does Feeling Safe Mean to You?

What has brought you to my book? What does feeling safe mean to you?

Something has drawn you to my book and I wonder what that is.

Each of us has a different relationship with feeling safe. In the course of writing this book, I asked many people to consider what 'feeling safe' meant to them.

Some talked about relationships with family, friends, neighbours. Many talked about stable jobs, having money in the bank, a roof over their heads. And of course, at the time of writing the final version of my book during the Covid-19 pandemic, many people talked about whether they felt safe to leave their houses, wear a mask, not wear a mask, hug other people, have the vaccine, hug people who'd had the vaccine. The issue of feeling safe was inescapable!

Some didn't know and couldn't answer the question. Others said the question made them feel profoundly uncomfortable, maybe even a bit sad. Often these were the ones who were not able to send me a response.

From Outside In, to Inside Out

I surveyed a group of people on social media – Trauma Thrivers they called themselves – and their answers were very revealing. This group of people had suffered extreme traumas and adversity, but they had come through it and no longer considered themselves to be victims of what they'd experienced. They considered themselves to be true thrivers.

Unlike most of the people I surveyed their focus was primarily on how they were feeling inside. They didn't seem to be as concerned about what was happening in their external world. The state of their inner world seemed to be what was most important rather than what was happening in their external world. It was as if they had been through so many traumas in their life that they had been forced to find a deeper sense of inner safety in order to thrive. Many of them also said they had a strong sense of being connected to something other than themselves and their external world and this was a significant source of safety for them.

Many people look outside of themselves for safety. It has become their normal way of being, their *modus operandi* – wake up in the morning, reach for the phone, what lies ahead in the day? What is happening in the world? Can I keep up? Am I good enough? How do I compare?

Safety has become externalized. Out there. We rely on the news or social media feed to tell us how to feel. We've forgotten how to be with ourselves, with quiet mornings, simply receiving the information coming from our own bodies, minds, hearts . . . we've forgotten how to listen.

Inside Out Versus Outside In

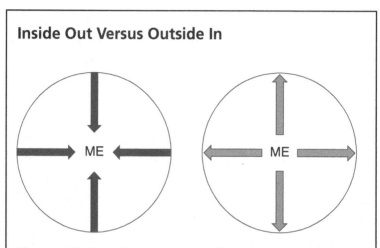

Figure 1.3 Outside in versus inside out approach to dealing with life.

When we respond to life from outside in, we end up simply *reacting* to life. What is happening *out there* determines how we feel *in here*, what we will do next, how we will think and behave, whether or not we will feel safe. In reality we have very little choice over what happens out there in the world and so we become victims of our environment and the world (See Figure 1.3).

Shifting the focus and responding to life from inside out – like the trauma thrivers, like I did in Brisbane all of those years ago, enables us to *respond* to life. We tap into a wellspring of resource and strength and this pathway, when travelled enough times, becomes our route to feeling safe. This re-routing isn't just a psychological or spiritual process, it is embedded in the nervous system. It is only when we understand and befriend our nervous system that we can find true inner safety.

Reflection Exercise: Embark on Your Journey

I urge you to consider your relationship with feeling safe and what it means to you. And in doing so, please be kind with yourself because you may stir up some feelings. That's normal.

I invite you to complete this exercise now. I suggest that you light a candle or sit in nature as you read these words. A notebook and pen beside you to journal your reflections and insights would be a good idea too.

With your eyes open or closed, reflect on these questions.

- What does feeling safe mean to me?
- How do I know when I am feeling safe?
- When have I recently felt really safe?
- What was I doing?
- Had something just happened or was it just a feeling that came over me?

Don't worry if you find these questions difficult to answer. It might be helpful to keep coming back to them as you progress through this book. For now, it might be enough to simply keep them in mind.

I want to take you into a deep journey with yourself. Consider what might support you as you read these words and do this work.

You could even gather support around you – maybe a friend or a group of like-minded individuals – who will go on this journey with you.

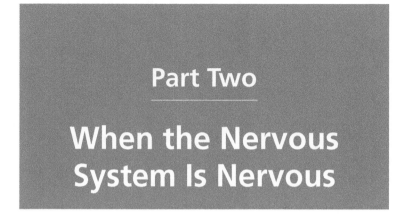

Part Two

When the Nervous System Is Nervous

Working With the Intelligence of Your Nervous System to Find Inner Safety

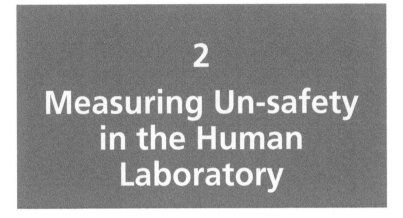

2
Measuring Un-safety in the Human Laboratory

'A quest for safety is the basis for living a successful life.'
—Stephen Porges, *The Polyvagal Theory*, 2017

Skewed Measurements

'Why are these people walking around as if they're ready to do battle?'

This was the question I asked my boss Malcolm more than 20 years ago. Wearing a white lab coat and working in a dingy basement clinic in Moorgate, I was measuring the health of City professionals – bankers, lawyers, accountants, insurers, chauffeurs, and office administrators.

Many of them seemed to have something in common.

Their bodies seemed to be working hard to help them keep up and this was reflected in the data I was recording on my white clipboard. The tests we were doing indicated that these human beings were stressed and running in survival mode. Their breathing patterns were shallow and restricted, electrocardiogram (ECG) traces and blood pressure showing signs of physiological stress; blood and body fat levels were high. In fact, in those days, my fellow physiologists and me coined the phrase 'trunkal thickening' to diplomatically describe the laying down of fat around the mid-section of the body – the proverbial plate of armour. Research shows that stress causes the elevation in levels of cortisol which leads to the laying down of abdominal fat and increased blood fats – cholesterol and triglycerides[*] – the body's way of armouring against stress.

All of the data was painting a picture of an urban hunter-gatherer who was working hard to overcome stress. Often, these people were hard to engage with, they seemed to be living in a different time zone, the future. They were impatient, driven, thinking about the next thing that needed to be done. Just not *here*, in the present.

This was the first time I really became aware of a mismatch between what I had expected to see from my theoretical studies and what I was measuring in practice. Measuring life in the human laboratory was a little different to measuring it in tissue culture plates and test tubes.

---

[*]Epel, E. et al. (2000). Stress and body shape: stress-induced cortisol secretion is consistently greater among women with central fat. *Psychosomatic Medicine* 62 (5): 623–632.

I became interested in what was happening in the milieu of the environment of these human beings that their physiology was behaving in this intelligent way. Because I want you to understand that our physiology *is* intelligent; it reads our environment and responds accordingly. This is the role of our autonomic nervous system (ANS) as I described at the beginning of my book – safe or unsafe?

So, what was happening out there in our world at that time? I began paying attention to what was happening in the world of the urban hunter-gatherer.

A Changing World – Speed, Noise, Demand, Technology

The World Wide Web had arrived, large brick-like mobile phones, email and inboxes, and everyone was speeding up to keep pace. We were no longer marching to the drumbeat of our own natural rhythms and physiology but rather to a manic beat of 'do more in less time, speed up, keep up!' I began running popular workshops in law and other professional services firms called 'Managing the Pace'.

In his book *Faster*, James Gleick described how the acceleration of time was stretching us all to our limits psychologically, neurologically, and physiologically – and I was measuring this first hand in my laboratory.

Often, I was seeing this 'skewed' data in young people who were supposedly fit and healthy, whose lives were secure in many respects – they had good, well-paid jobs, strong relationships, beautiful homes, and social networks. So why were they physiologically arming themselves as if they were about to do battle?

And what has this got to do with feeling unsafe? This is where my interest was becoming peeked.

I knew (and know) that our physiology and entire nervous system is designed along the premise of SAFE or UNSAFE.

Our autonomic nervous system is the vital system that regulates all involuntary physiological processes such as heart rate, blood pressure, digestion, respiration, sexual function, rest, and sleep. It also enables us to fight threat if we perceive ourselves to be unsafe.

So, we respond *in here* according to how we perceive the world *out there*. This is nothing to do with whether objectively the world is safe or unsafe. It all boils down to one simple perception:

Does my nervous system feel my environment to be safe or unsafe?

Now this is a bit of a conundrum because where we come unstuck is when we *think* we're safe but our body *feels* unsafe. The illusion of safety.

This is what I was measuring in the living laboratory – a quickening in our external world that was stretching us, driving us to try to keep up, resulting in a somatic** experience that we had no direct control over – at least not at that time, as it took at least a decade for the yoga, mindfulness, meditation, and wellness world to gain some traction.

So, here we have a simple situation of safe people who feel unsafe *in their bodies*. They *know* they're safe but they *feel* unsafe. It starts as a distant rumble as we accelerate to keep pace. Impatience and multitasking become the norm and the body – intelligently – begins to behave as if it's constantly gearing up deal with threat. And this becomes the norm.

But the problem lies in a disconnect between the Thinking Brain and the Feeling Body.

We can think one thing. But feel another. Our clever, rational, intellectual mind tells us 'This is OK, I'll get through this, I can do it' but our bodies are registering something else. And that something else bubbles up at night, when we return to that childlike state that we go to in sleep, when our defences are down. Stored sensations in the body rise up in our consciousness – usually at some point between 2 a.m. and 4 a.m. Sometimes it hits as soon as we put our head on the pillow and the body sensations trigger the 'mad monkey' – that voice in

---

**Somatic – meaning related to the body rather than the mind.

our brain that yacks away telling us we're not safe, reinforcing the bodily sensations of being in survival mode.

Until we begin to understand and navigate the workings of our nervous system, we are trapped in this mismatch of what we feel we should be doing and thinking and how we are feeling deeply in the body.

The real work lies in understanding and befriending our nervous system. It also lies in understanding the real roots of how we develop inner safety – how it is rooted in our childhood, and even before that when we grew in our mother's belly, and before that too way back into our ancestry. Feeling safe goes back far into our history and it goes deep.

You will now learn about the physiology of safety – 'the science of feeling safe enough to fall in love with life and take risks' as Deb Dana describes it. My belief is that when we understand what is happening in our bodies, why it is happening, and then, importantly, what we can do to navigate our responses to life, this is when we can achieve true life empowerment.

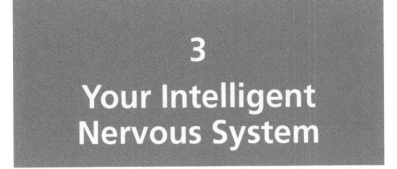

3
Your Intelligent Nervous System

'The great thing, then, in all education, is to make our nervous system our ally instead of our enemy.'
—William James, *Habit*

Introduction to the Key Principles of Safety Science

What you will now read is, arguably, one of the most important sections of this book. This is where you learn about the science of feeling safe. I urge you not to gloss over or skip this chapter – I want you to gain a clear understanding of how our physiology responds to feeling safe or not safe. More importantly, I want you to leave this section with a clear understanding of how *you* react to the world and the daily challenges it presents you with for, armed with this self-awareness, you will then be able to make the choices that enable you to thrive.

In writing this chapter, I have attempted to make accessible the brilliant work of Stephen Porges and Deb Dana. To this end, I will introduce you to the following key safety science concepts:

- The three branches of the Autonomic Nervous System involved in enabling us to stay safe.
- How and why these three branches evolved in a particular evolutionary timeline and how they play out in everyday life.
- Pendulation and regulation – how we are meant to move back and forth between the three branches of our nervous system in normal life in order to regulate our physiology and thrive, and what happens when we don't.
- Neuroception – how we sense the world around us.
- Interoception – that less well-known sense that helps us to understand what is happening in our body.
- Social engagement – how we engage with the world around us to create safe, trustworthy, and loving connections.
- Epigenetics – here I hope to show you how our relationship with safety goes deep, perhaps deeper than you might have imagined. How we show up in the world today, and how we will do so in the future, is a function of what came before us – our birth experiences, your mother's experience as she carried you in her belly, and even the experiences of your forefathers have left an imprint in your nervous system which can play out in your 'today

world', sometimes in a way that might seem illogical or confusing – why am I reacting this way? Doing the work on healing your relationship with feeling safe might involve going back so that you can move forward with the strength and conviction you need in order to thrive.

A Day in the Life Of

Scenario 1: She wakes to the violent clamour of her mobile phone alarm clock. Deliberately set to awaken her assertively, non-negotiably. It has to be that way as she's so tired these days. She groans, grabs her phone, and puts it on snooze. The second clamour seems to happen just microseconds later and this time there's no snoozing. The alarm off, she lies – just a few minutes – phone in hand while casting her mind over her day ahead. She's already out there in the world even though her body hasn't yet left the bed. Have to do's, must do's, should do's flooding in. Her body tenses, her stomach knots and queases – no time or inclination for breakfast this morning, time to get going.

Rush to the train station, compete – unsuccessfully – to get a seat. Standing the whole journey again, pressed up against people she doesn't want to be pressed up against. Work is manic. Back-to-back meetings and lunch grabbed at her desk while working through emails. She leaves work at 6 p.m. and tiredness means plans to go the gym are on hold again. It's Friday, maybe she'll go at some point over the weekend. Crash out exhausted on the sofa with a takeaway and a glass of wine. She feels fed up and somewhat hopeless about the never-ending treadmill of her life.

Scenario 2: I'm sitting on a fallen log overhanging the river where I love to swim throughout the year, legs dangling in, enjoying the pleasant cool of the water on a warm summer's day. Not too hot. Just perfect. Mira, my rescue puppy sniffing around happily, running up and down the slippery tree trunk, showing off for me, as she does. I'm listening to a podcast – appropriately, Richard Powers' *Overstory*, the deservedly Pulitzer-Prize-winning book about man's relationship with trees and nature. All is well in my world.

In seconds this situation changes.

Mira slips on the log. I reach forward to grab her. My phone dislodges from its snug place in my back pocket. Plop! I hear. I can no longer hear Powers' voice.

The spiteful river has been taken my phone. Just seconds before beloved, now I hate her.

Shock.

Disbelief.

Heart and mind racing. Mouth dry. Can't breathe. Can't make myself breathe. Nausea. Overwhelm – unable to receive well-meaning advice.

Panic! Someone – anyone – please help me!

Self-recrimination, guilt, shame (How could I have been so stupid? Why did I? Why didn't I?).

Grief and sorrow – what have I lost? Can any of it be salvaged?

Realization.

Numbness. Can't think straight.

More realization. Calm. Problem solving. Seeing opportunities. Coming to terms. Feeling safe.

I describe these two scenarios. The first, a common way of starting the day for so many people. The second, an occurrence that took place just a few days ago when I lost my phone, irretrievably, in the river by my home. Both illustrate how the nervous system can become nervous.

What both have in common is that thoughts generated in the mind and in response to things that can happen in everyday life have caused the nervous system disequilibrium. There's no masked attacker, hairy mammoth, or sabre-toothed tiger.

In scenario 1 – what lies in store for me? How will I keep up? There's too much! I can't cope with it – I have to try harder. The physiological response to ongoing and constant demand is created more insidiously than the short, sharp shock of the incident of a drowned mobile phone. There are the demands that sit in the inbox, there's the fear generated by news headlines and reports, there's the constant pressure of social media. And of course, there's the self-generated, perfectionistic, imposter syndrome fearing internal demand to lean in, keep up with a relentless workload, be the best.

In scenario 2 – again, the mind (my mind) creating feelings of un-safety. How will I survive without my phone? Am I alone in the world? Who do I now have in my life?

It might sound far-fetched but for a while (a couple of hours or so) I'm embarrassed to say that the loss of my phone felt like an existential crisis. I felt *unsafe*. I felt unmoored, untethered, lost. At the time, I knew I was overreacting, but the phone had come to *mean something* to me at a time when I was alone and had been for over a year. During the isolation of the pandemic, it had become something of a lifeline. I received daily messages – often voice notes from caring friends – and I felt less alone. I *knew* logically, intellectually, that what had happened was not a catastrophe, but my body was reacting in a different way – as if it was under threat.

And in fact, I went through the seven classic stages of the grief cycle:

• Shock and denial.
• Pain and guilt
• Disbelief and numbness

- Anger and bargaining
- Depression
- The upward turn
- Reconstruction and working through
- Acceptance and hope.

There are real threats and there are imagined threats. Problems arise when we start to *feel* as if the life we're living is threatening to our survival. This book isn't called *Think Safe*, it's called *Finding Inner Safety*. The ability to *feel* safe is about acknowledging and working with the *embodied* experience. If we take the incident of my phone, I knew that I was safe and that this annoying (and expensive) mishap was in no way a threat to my survival but my initial physiological response was heightened and adrenalized. Once the embodied response had been worked through (I will tell you how to do that later), I reached a place of calm and acceptance – and even opportunity as, for the next three days, I enjoyed the feelings of peace and simplicity that came from not having a phone.

Whatever it is, wherever it comes from, we are – or rather our nervous system is – constantly scanning our environment, looking for risk, managing risk, and creating patterns of connection or disconnection by changing our physiological state. Our nervous system is the surveillance system that constantly scans our environment sending messages to the brain. These messages are then translated by the brain into beliefs that guide our daily living.

As the nineteenth-century grandfather of psychology, William James said: 'The greatest thing then, in all education, is to make our nervous system our ally as opposed to our enemy.'

When you befriend your nervous system, you acquire choice. You learn to listen and then choose. Herein lies freedom. In the listening, there needs to be understanding. You listen and then you can ask yourself the following questions:

- What does this mean?
- What is it telling me?
- How do I want to react?
- Do I have a choice to do something differently and do I want to?

This is the conscious path to finding and strengthening inner safety.

Let me now help you to understand your amazing nervous system.

Polyvagal Theory (Viva Las Vagus!)

The way we react to life and perceive the world is governed by our nervous system, or rather, the Autonomic Nervous System (ANS). The vagus nerve is the main nerve of the ANS originating in the head and travelling through the body. In fact, it is called The Wanderer as it travels through the body regulating and controlling many important bodily functions, such as: breathing, heartbeat, appetite, immunity, sexual function, and digestion.

I now want to introduce you to the **Polyvagal Theory** that was discovered by the aforementioned Dr Stephen Porges in the 1990s. He would have elucidated his theory when I was a university student studying for my degree and then PhD in physiology. But back then we weren't told anything about Polyvagal Theory as it hadn't gained credibility as yet. It was more than 20 years later, when I was working on this book, trying to get things straight in my own mind, that I happened across Porges' work. An important part of the safety jigsaw puzzle fell into place – and not just for this book but in my own personal life, as I was able to make sense of the things I'd been through and how I'd responded to life.

Until I'd come across Polyvagal Theory, I was familiar with the idea of our autonomic nervous system being divided into a two-branched antagonistic system – the sympathetic nervous system (SNS) being the activated, stress hormone-driven part of the nervous system. The SNS responds to cues of danger, triggering the release of adrenaline and switching on the 'fight or flight' response. The other branch of the nervous system is the parasympathetic nervous system (PNS), also known as the rest and digest system or calming branch of the ANS. As I'd learnt about it, the PNS was involved in all vegetative, restorative functions – sleep, digestion, sexual function, immunity, and repair. My understanding was that, in daily life, we oscillate between these two branches of the nervous system, reacting according to our external world and in service of 'safe or unsafe?'

Porges identified another aspect to the nervous system. He discovered that the vagus nerve was in fact divided into two parts:

* The **ventral vagus** pathway, which responds to cues of safety, enables us to feel safe, enables us to build connection with others.
* The **dorsal vagus** pathway, which responds to cues of extreme threat and danger. We freeze, lose connection with others, lose awareness, become numb and dissociated.

So, now we see that there are three pathways for responding to the world.

1. **Ventral vagus** – I am safe to connect with life, I trust life, all is well in my world.
2. **Sympathetic nervous system** – I am unsafe and I don't trust this situation, I need to fight or flee.
3. **Dorsal vagus** – I feel extremely unsafe, I cannot bear this, I must disappear, if I play dead I might survive, I am powerless, I have no choice.

Note to reader: You might want to put the book down and pause for a moment, giving yourself an opportunity to reflect on the last few days when you might have cycled between these three parts of your nervous system.

When have you felt safe recently? What exactly were you doing? Did you feel **connected** to something or someone when you were having this experience?

When have you felt stressed and **activated** recently? Were you afraid or angry? Did you feel the impulse to do something drastic about it? It might even have been an email or text message that raised your hackles, or a driver who cut you up rudely on the road making you swear out loud and shake your fist at them!

Can you remember a time recently when you felt shut down, powerless, and **disconnected**? Maybe you were sitting in a meeting listening to someone saying something you really don't agree with but feeling unable to speak up? Or a moment when something happened that was so overwhelming that you couldn't react or felt numb with shock?

If I relate this to my drowned mobile phone incident, I can see clearly how I cycled through all three nervous system responses, initially feeling the shocked numbness of the dorsal vagus, followed by feeling somewhat annoyed with myself for not having done a variety of things that could have stopped the incident. And then I moved quickly to action to try to salvage the situation, phoning the mobile phone company, arranging for a new SIM card to be sent to me, contacting those I could contact and letting them know I'd be uncontactable by mobile phone for a while. I was spurred into action by my sympathetic nervous system! And then a sense of calm acceptance descended on me, and I actually enjoyed the peace that came from not being at the beck and call of my device – my ventral vagus was fired up and working.

Evolution of Our Nervous System

Stephen Porges' work showed that there is an evolutionary timeline to the development of these three aspects of the nervous system and our nervous system intelligently decides which pathway to use, depending on how we perceive our environment.

The dorsal vagus evolved first so it's our oldest nervous system pathway – the reptilian branch of the ANS. It probably evolved so that our ancient vertebrate ancestors could 'play dead' and immobilize to survive threat. This part of the nervous system ticks away in the background, maintaining the basic operational functioning of the body. I view it as being a bit like the disk operating system (DOS) that normally runs the basic utilities of a computer for our body. It keeps us alive but not particularly engaged with life – the lights are on but no one's home.

Then came the sympathetic nervous system and the ability to mobilize to fight threat.

The ventral vagus pathway is the most recently evolved part of the nervous system, uniquely designed in mammals to enable social engagement, connection (see Figure 3.1).

The Evolutionary Timeline of Nervous System Development

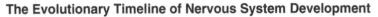

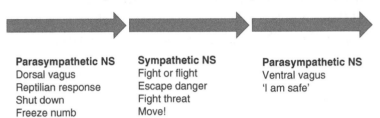

Parasympathetic NS	**Sympathetic NS**	**Parasympathetic NS**
Dorsal vagus	Fight or flight	Ventral vagus
Reptilian response	Escape danger	'I am safe'
Shut down	Fight threat	
Freeze numb	Move!	
'I must not move'		

Figure 3.1 Diagram of evolutionary timeline.

So, when we feel safe in our world, we are grounded in the ventral vagus, calm, peaceful, and happy to connect with other human beings. Shock, stress, and danger can send us backwards on the evolutionary timeline into the sympathetic nervous system (take action!) or even further back into the dorsal vagus in which we immobilize and shut down to survive.

In everyday life we **pendulate** back and forth between these nervous system states – engaging and connecting, activating and mobilizing, and disconnecting. We need each part of our intelligent nervous system as they enable us to respond to life and to survive. Even our shutdown nervous system, the dorsal vagus, has its place as it helps us to survive horrendous shocks and onslaughts and not feel it, and thus survive. But it is important that there is a normal healthy cycling back and forth between social engagement and activation/mobilization. Every physiological process runs on this basic principle of pendulation or contraction and expansion – the heartbeat, our breathing, the sleep–wake cycle, body temperature control. This pulsing is the basic principle of life too, seen in the ebb and flow of ocean tides, the opening and closing of birds' wings in flight. Pendulation is necessary for us to thrive in life, to grow, to rest and sleep, to respond and react to other human beings, to live healthily and optimally (See Figure 3.2).

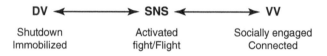

Figure 3.2 Nervous system pendulation.

Regulation, Co-regulation, Dysregulation

Moving back and forth between these different branches of the nervous system enables us to navigate in the world. This is called **self-regulation.** We **co-regulate** in our relationships with others; when we form healthy connections, express warm and authentic feelings towards each other. So here, there is regulation being brought about as we interact with others, and it makes us feel safe, trusting, as if we belong.

Co-regulation is seen at its most essential when a child is born. The baby initially lacks the ability to fend for itself, to feel safe on its own. The mother–baby connection creates a mutual bond of co-regulation. The mother's facial expressions, voice, and gestures calm and soothe the baby, taking it into the ventral vagus state, and this has the reciprocal effect of calming the mother.

Dysregulation arises when we are relating to someone or a situation that we don't trust. We start to feel a stirring of something in our body that we can't control. There are situations in which it might be appropriate to raise our hackles (sympathetic activation) or withdraw and stay quiet (dorsal vagus) but in the dysregulated state, our physiological response starts to feel beyond our control. For example, an extreme sympathetic activation state might be having a panic attack or flying into a violent rage. Plummeting uncontrollably into a dorsal vagus state could show up as feeling utterly hopeless and suicidal.

The ability to self-regulate in our relationships is vital to being able to thrive. As human beings we are designed to connect and build healthy relationships with other people – this is key to our health and vitality on every level – physical, emotional, mental, and spiritual.

Can you think back to a recent time where you were with someone else, and you started to feel uncomfortable in your body? Or maybe you felt a great sense of ease come over you as you talked with this person. Can you think of the people in your life with whom you feel at ease, peaceful, open, and trusting? And there may be times when, even with these people, you have moments where it feels uncomfortable between you. Maybe you say something, and the air is cleared and suddenly you feel at ease again. This is life, and the safer we feel in ourselves to show who we are, be who we are, say what we need to say, the greater the chance we can self-regulate in the face of challenging circumstances.

Habituation to Survival – A Nervous System Perspective

Problems arise when we become *stuck in survival mode*, as I have already described in this book. When we become immobilized by life, feeling powerless in circumstances over which we feel we have no control, or if we become stuck in hypervigilance, constantly leaned in to life feeling we can't stop, we can't rest, addicted to busyness. We haven't evolved to move efficiently between shutdown and social engagement or shutdown and activation.

When we are stuck in the dorsal vagus system it can become a way of defence in life. Many people become depressed, hopeless, chronically exhausted, and sick because they are trapped in the immobilization circuit.

On the other hand, and as I have described before, some people habituate to living in sympathetic nervous system overdrive. They can't stop, always busy, always on the go. The stress hormones, adrenaline, noradrenaline, and cortisol, when depleted, are supplemented with caffeine and dopamine hits from their electronic devices – anything to keep them in 'doing' mode. Running in this part of the nervous system is not sustainable and I have worked with many people who eventually crashed into the burnout patterns of chronic fatigue, adrenal exhaustion, or other health crises, life forcing them to 'rest' in the immobilization mode of the dorsal vagus.

Another pattern I'm seeing a lot is where dorsal vagus immobilization shows up as the inability to express or speak one's truth. Words unspoken become locked into the body, often in the neck and shoulders causing headaches and migraines or held tightly in the gut giving rise to digestive disorders and irritable bowel syndrome.

For example, Anita was a compulsive 'good girl'. She had always behaved herself and her parents couldn't even remember her having tantrums as a child. Quiet and studious, she always did well at school, just quietly getting on with it. When she was 10 years old, she started having frequent severe migraines and suffered from bruxism, nocturnal grinding of teeth that was so extreme that she had to wear a mouth guard while sleeping. The first time I saw her, I felt she had a classic pattern of immobilization despite her somewhat impassive smile. All of her life she hadn't felt safe to express herself, keeping her jaw clamped shut tight and her words and feelings locked in. A highly creative artist, her symptoms started to ease when she began to express herself through her art and painting. She covered the canvas in ferocious gothic art but, at last, she had found the safety to express.

I saw this again recently when I worked online with Amanda, a 31-year-old management consultant who had been referred to me by her company's human resources department. She had been signed off from work because she was exhausted and was no longer able to maintain the gruelling hours she'd been working before being referred to me. Again, at our first meeting I was struck by the lack of expression on her face. She smiled but it was as if she felt she had to and often her smiles didn't reach her eyes at all – they seemed dead and expressionless, the classic picture of dorsal vagus freeze.

Sensing Our Inner and Outer World

How do we read what is happening out there in the world? How do we decide what is safe and what isn't?

Years ago, when I didn't know much about the science of safety, I really didn't understand why there were times when I would walk into an environment – often a corporate environment – and just feel uncomfortable. I didn't realize then that my nervous system was giving me information about the space I'd entered. I just knew that I liked visiting some of my clients' offices more than others! Joining the dots, I later realized that often the feelings I experienced – an unaccustomed tightening in my stomach or wave of anxiety in my solar plexus – were related to the culture of that organization. Some of these big chrome and glass buildings housed organizations that were driven and fear-filled. These were the environments in which there was a high incidence of burnout, high stress levels, and mental health problems. Often, they were classic Type A* environments in which employees felt they needed to perform in a certain way in order to get ahead. To my body, these environments felt 'unsafe' on some level, even though I was enjoying the work I was doing and on a rational level, knew I wasn't walking into a den of sabre-toothed tigers when I entered their revolving doors.

Conversely, there are many environments that I love visiting. I have been teaching on leadership programmes at Ashridge Business School for many years. My drive there takes around an hour and a half and a lot of that is on London's wonderful M25 motorway. In the last 10 minutes or so of the journey, I drive through Ashridge Forest and I feel my shoulders drop and my nervous

---

*Type A personalities tend to be driven, competitive, aggressive, and perfectionistic individuals. Derived from the work of cardiologists Friedman and Rosenman in 1976 who showed that people with such personality traits have a greater cardiac risk than type Bs, who tend to be more patient, laid back, and considered in their approach to life. The theory has since been disproved but the principles still apply when describing individuals and environments that are characterized by an exaggerated sense of urgency and stress.

system settles. Walking into the famous stately home that houses the business school (and the place where the famous moving staircase scene from the Harry Potter movie was filmed) I feel even more ease entering my body and mind – the perfect state of regulation in which I can deliver my presentations to leaders from all around the world.

Maybe because of the environment I was brought up in, I am finely tuned and sensitive. But I also believe that many people are sensitive, but they are used to ignoring the whispers of their bodies, shutting out (or in) uncomfortable sensations – and sometimes we just need to get on with it, don't we?

We are like trees sensing the world. Our antennae are like the leaves and branches, waving in the wind, feeding information back to the trunk and then down deep into our roots. But what are our actual antennae?

The autonomic nervous system responds to the environment around us via a process called **neuroception**. Neuroception is our sensing of the environment around us with our senses – sight, sound, smell, touch – far *below the level of our conscious awareness*. So, there is an important distinction here: perception is what we *consciously* detect and evaluate, neuroception is what we automatically and reflexively evaluate in our environment without awareness.

One of the sleep hygiene tips I often impart to my clients is that your bedroom should feel like a sanctuary. Remember, we sleep when we feel safe. So, you should walk into your bedroom and the sight, sound, and smell of your sleep space should make you feel at ease, comforted, safe to sleep. This is neuroception at play.

Our neuroceptive abilities are the antennae of our nervous system. They give you your gut feeling, they tell you whether you've walked into a room of people that feels good or not. They tell you whether you're safe or unsafe, whether someone feels trustworthy or not. You know when you just walk into a space and get a feeling about it?

So, we receive these signals from the antennae, and the ANS makes a judgement, assesses the risk – safe or unsafe? Depending on the answer to this assessment, signals are routed along one of the three pathways described above – connect, mobilize, or immobilize?

Interoception is the process by which we make sense of the sensations taking place in our body. It is how we 'compute' in our minds that which is happening in our bodies. Do you remember when I described in my own personal journey the distortion between feeling excited and feeling afraid? In my mind they had become muddled, and a big part of my healing journey was to learn how to make sense of what I was feeling and to place the correct interpretations on the sensations.

Meanings Matter

There is another important consideration here, another overlay to how our nervous system goes about sensing, responding, and trying to keep us safe and that is to do with the *meaning* attached to the event or occurrence.

If we go right back to the personal story I shared at the beginning – the losing of my mobile phone – my perception of the situation was, OK, this is a pain in the neck, an inconvenience, but there's no threat to my existence. However, for a couple of hours, my body was having a different reaction – it was in shock because of what my phone, slightly unbeknown to me, had come to represent. In a time of isolation and loneliness, it had become a major source of connection with friends, with my mother in South America, my daily phone calls with my daughter, my work which I love and had also become another source of meaning and purpose during these difficult times. Because of what it meant to me my body reacted in shock and shut down.

In the hours after the loss, I was able to make contact with my daughter, a kindly neighbour offered a spare phone, I called my mother on my landline phone (yes I still have one!). I'd known all along that all was well in my world but my nervous system needed time to catch up.

Initially – and a day or so after the event – I was a tad embarrassed when I thought about how I had reacted. However, when I later processed, without judgement, what had happened and why my nervous system had reacted in this way I was able to make sense of my reaction.

We are constantly evaluating and assessing our environment through the lenses of meaning and history!

Meaning: In other words, what did the mobile phone mean to me at the time I'd lost it? It had come to represent connection and belonging in a time of isolation.

History: It had also deeply triggered feelings of loss and abandonment which were embedded in my nervous system from childhood, from past relationships, from my sister's sudden death, and from a recent loss that took place during the pandemic.

Social Engagement (and Wearing Masks)

As I write this book, we are – hopefully – emerging from the Covid-19 pandemic. One of the biggest impacts of this global pandemic, aside from the loss of human life, has been the loneliness and mental ill-health wrought by lockdown, self-isolation, and the wearing of masks. This isn't a commentary on the rights and wrongs of mask wearing nor a judgement on their efficacy as a method of reducing the spread of infection, but rather a reflection on the impact on our ability to connect and relate to each other during a time when we've really needed – perhaps more than ever – to comfort and reassure each other.

To help you to understand my point, let me tell you about how we are designed to engage with and bond with each other. I've already described the co-regulation that takes place when a child bonds with its mother and vice versa. Stephen Porges also added to safety science the concept of **social engagement**, the process whereby we bond with others by:

Talking or vocalisation – we listen to the intonation in the voice and the **vocal prosody** which is the rhythm, stress, and intonation of speech, and this creates safety (or not). The mother's voice speaks lulling, soft, and soothing tones which calm the baby's nervous system. But even for adults, the right vocal prosody helps us to engage with the other, trust them, choose to connect or walk away. During the pandemic, when all of my speaking engagements were switched to online events, despite the fact that I'd been presenting online for over a decade, I became even more aware of the need to modulate my voice to build trust, keep the attendees engaged and listening so they didn't leave. Sometimes, all they could see was my slides and they could hear my voice, which made it even more challenging, as when we see the face of the other, it also builds trust (or not).

Facial expressions and gestures – the muscles around the eyes that are engaged in smiling are called the *orbicularis oculi*. They were discovered in 1862 by the French anatomist Duchenne de Boulogne, who said that these were the muscles that are engaged in a 'real' happy smile as opposed to the 'fake' happy smile. This is when the smile reaches the eyes. Other key facial muscles involved in building true connection are the muscles around the mouth – the *zygomaticus major and minor* along with the *levator labii superioris* muscles. These muscles are connected to facial nerves which let the brain know when we are smiling, truly smiling. When we smile and contract these muscles, the nerve signalling to the brain stimulates the production of the pain-relieving hormones, endorphins. We also produce the so-called love and trust hormone, oxytocin. Again, fake smiling doesn't do this.

So, nature has anatomically designed us with a set of apparatus to build trusting relationships and connections, all key to feeling safe. But how does this work in the world we inhabit today, with all of its current challenges and, in particular, the virtual world?

All Alone Together

Years ago, when I began delivering virtual presentations, I became aware that I needed to work even more on being grounded and safe within myself in order to bring that through in my voice and facial expression, so I could convey that through the electronic medium, inducing safety and trust to my audiences. A lot of it was instinctive but I focused harder on voice modulation and, when they could see me, my facial expressions and hand gestures.

Sometimes, if the session was only audio-based, I would close my eyes while presenting and try to 'feel' into my audience as if I could somehow connect with them more deeply this way. I was less concerned with the slides if I was using them, and I wanted to interact with my audiences as much possible, getting them to interact with me using chat functions rather than doing polls. I ensured that I was feeling as grounded in my body as possible, making sure that I was well rested and exercised, I'd eaten and hydrated well. I made a point of feeling my feet on the ground throughout my presentations (more about this later) and breathing deep into my belly whenever I could.

As someone who has been doing public speaking for a long time, I have long understood the importance of 'state preparation' and being steady in myself in order to not only present at my best but also create greater feelings of safety and trust in my audiences. I've noticed that when I'm feeling safe in myself, my audiences are more likely to open up and share. My state affects theirs. This was particularly brought home to me when recently, while delivering a presentation on stress and perfectionism to more than a hundred people from an investment bank, the Wi-Fi connection failed five times during the presentation due to network problems in my neighbourhood. Each time this happened I was forced to leave the presentation and dial back in. Eventually, I had to turn off my camera to maximize whatever connection I did have, so they could hear me but not see me. The irony was not lost on me. I felt my frustration building and stress levels rising – I am a reformed perfectionist, by the way – but worked even harder at staying safe and holding on to my audience. I told them how I was feeling and what I was doing to maintain my state of regulation. In the end, the session went so well that the HR manager called me straight afterwards to reassure me of the positive feedback. Not only this, but she later told me that, as a result of the feedback from this session more than six hundred people had signed up for the next session!

In this online world we live in today, we have to work to find even greater inner safety because when we exude it, other people feel it. Years ago, while studying psychiatry and psychology part-time at London's Guys Hospital, I wrote an essay entitled 'The Difference Between True Relating and Mere Interactions'. This was in the late nineties and the technology storm hadn't quite landed in our world full force . . . but it was rumbling. Back then, I predicted that we would need to work on our connections more consciously and mindfully in order to build and maintain cohesion and trust in a world where communication was increasingly becoming remote and electronic. At the time, the notion of 'feeling safe' wasn't at all on my radar; it was at least another decade before it came into range.

It was at the psychiatric clinic, where once I'd been a patient, that my interest in safety was piqued. I was talking a lot about the influence of technology and got involved in setting up the clinic's first adolescent technology addiction clinic. The idea of people, and especially young people, becoming addicted to gaming and gambling was, in the opinion of some people, extreme but the media was quick to jump on the bandwagon 'we're all addicted to technology' which I didn't agree with at all, but I did feel that we were all – myself included – becoming overly dependent on our devices (I remind you of my extreme reaction to losing my phone!).

Sherry Turkle, in her book *Alone Together* writes about the loneliness and frightening rise in mental health problems facing young people because of their reliance on their electronic devices for communicating with each other. At the time of writing this book, the incidence in teenagers aged between 14 and 19 years, of self-harming, suicide, drug usage, risk-taking behaviours, and behavioural and mental health disorders such as psychosis, anxiety, and depression is at an alarming level and rising. My 17-year-old daughter tells me how she has decided to remove all social media apps from her phone. The pressure to be included – to engage, to keep up with, to be more popular than, to be constantly plugged in – had created so much stress and unhappiness that she and many of her friends have decided to disconnect. Even for these 'digital natives' the way in which they communicate with each other does not easily build safety and trust – rapid-fire 'likes' and emojis, text talk and phone language. Are they truly relating or merely interacting? My daughter tells me that a popular way of invalidating someone else's importance is to refer to them as 'irrelevant' or to 'ghost' them – just shut them off, don't reply, or reply with minimal characters and a full stop.

'Are you going to Amber's party tonight?'

'Yh.' (Meaning 'yeah')

Minimal interaction. You're not worth more. You are unimportant and irrelevant.

This is the world our children are growing up in and the impact on their nervous systems cannot be underplayed, particularly when we consider the distressing mental health statistics. My belief, and concern, is that the way in which young people have come to rely on technology as the architect of their relationships is creating mental illness – a dysfunctional pendulation between sympathetic nervous system activation and dorsal vagus shutdown. When we are living from our dorsal vagus we feel disempowered, immobilized, frozen, and stuck in bad feelings. Anna, a 16-year-old who has been self-harming for more than a year said: 'When I feel like this, it feels so bad and I want do anything to feel something, to feel better.' This is when she cuts herself.

Peter Levine, a long-time friend and colleague of Porges, studied the shutdown response through animal observations and bodywork with clients. In *Waking the Tiger: Healing Trauma*, he explained that emerging from shutdown requires a shudder or shake to discharge suspended fight-or-flight energy. In a life-threatening situation, if we have shutdown and an opportunity for active survival presents itself, we can wake ourselves up. But the reality of life is that our adolescents, when faced with with the 'threat' presented by social media, the feelings of irrelevance and unimportance, don't find it so easy to shake off. Not surprisingly, too many people turn to risk-taking and harmful behaviours as a means of escaping the powerlessness of dorsal vagus shutdown.

And it's not just the younger generation which suffers. Is it really possible to build true connection when it has become the norm that communication these days takes place amidst multitasking, talking to someone while looking at virtual others on laptops and other electronic devices?

A few years ago, I was delivering a workshop on resilience and 'leading from the centre' to a small group of senior management consultants. The firm they worked for was successful and driven, with highly perfectionistic employees, a strong work ethic of 'the client comes first', and a high rate of burnout. During the half-day workshop, one of my key messages was that in order to be an inspired leader and to create strong, bonded teams, one has to be the change, to demonstrate self-care behaviours that team members feel enabled to follow themselves. I was also planning to engage them in a conversation in which we could talk about the importance of authentic communication for building connection and cohesion.

When I walked into the room to begin the session, only half of them were there and they were deeply engrossed in their inboxes. I greeted them and a couple said a half-hearted hello without looking up. The others ignored me and continued tap-tapping away at their keyboards. The session started and a few still hadn't turned up and when they did, they continued looking at their phones and laptops! I repeated my opening request that everyone put their electronic devices away and that I would be timetabling breaks when they could check their messages, but my request was ignored. Occasionally, someone would leave the room while I was mid-sentence to take or make a call.

And how did I feel? At first, angry and frustrated, my sympathetic nervous system on high alert, adrenaline coursing through my body. I challenged their behaviours, but my words were met with stony looks and lack of comprehension – didn't I understand how important they were? Eventually, I felt myself giving up and deciding that I would just make it to the end and leave. An old stammer resurfaced and my confidence began to dwindle. I felt irrelevant and without a voice. I left the session with a pounding headache and feeling exhausted and numb. I was in dorsal vagus shutdown. On my commute home I remember feeling cold and strangely disconnected from the world around me. When I arrived home, I just wanted to get into bed and sleep, but I forced myself go for a run along the river and in the rain. Feelings of anger resurfaced, and I gave them up to the pounding of my feet on the ground. The rain washed away my frustration and gave it to the river. I finished my run with resolve and conviction – I had returned.

I later arranged a call with the HR manager, and she said that the feedback from the session had not been positive. I explained what had happened and that I was not prepared to continue working on this leadership programme unless there was internal support from a senior partner and agreement on acceptable and unacceptable behaviours. For example, I felt it was unacceptable to be speaking to a group of people while they were looking at their laptops and phones. She said this was not something they could change as these senior managers were particularly busy. That was the last time I presented at the firm.

Reality Shows and Frozen 'Perfection'

Recently, my daughter and I watched an episode of a reality programme in which very wealthy women bickered and fought throughout the show. I couldn't quite work out what they were fighting over but it seemed to be dramatic. However, I could only tell this from the background music which was dramatic and suspense-building. The women's perfectly 'beautiful' faces were impassive and immobile as a result of the aesthetic work they'd had done to supposedly enhance their looks! Botox, fillers, and face-lifts resulted in complete absence of movement of the muscles around the eyes and mouth. The backing music was designed to inform the viewer of the emotional flavour of each scene – essential, as without this, the empty, expressionless faces of the characters gave nothing away. I found myself unsurprised that the women were constantly at war – how could they build genuine trust with each other when their faces revealed so little of what they were really feeling? Many of the women were in their forties and fifties but I've also seen other reality shows in which younger people – millennials and even teenagers – have had cosmetic surgery to 'enhance' their looks and, in the process, have ended up creating the same frozen, strangely perfect looks in which expressions cannot be read as the facial muscles are rendered immobile. Instagram and other social media platforms are similarly plastered with images of 'perfect' wrinkle-free, pouty-lipped faces in which appearances have been enhanced either through cosmetic surgery, make-up, or clever lighting and photography.

This is not a diatribe against having cosmetic surgery, but I believe that our society has become excessively wedded to the notion of perfection and image, to the detriment of authenticity, our ability to trust what we see, or, as Porges describes it, the 'misinterpretation of intentions'. And how does this relate to the nervous system? As Porges says, we need the ventral vagus cues to tell us whether we are safe in our relating to others – so we look at the facial expressions as well as listening to the voice. If the facial muscles are frozen, for example, with Botox in the upper face, then the expressions of joy and happiness are dampened . . . emotional responses are then misinterpreted.

Human beings are designed for connection; it is vital for our mental health and wellbeing, our very happiness. When we connect deeply and authentically, using the apparatus that we have evolved for this very purpose – our facial muscles, voices, our wrinkles, and genuine smiles – we settle and steady ourselves. We feel safe. During this ongoing pandemic, the need to put distance between ourselves and others, to not touch, to wear masks, has additionally created a great deal of loneliness as we are denied one of our most basic needs – the need to connect, *truly* connect.

Safety in Connection

I have always considered myself to have a strong introverted side to my nature, but as the pandemic wore on, the isolation and loneliness started to affect me too. Unusually, I found myself reaching out to connect with my local community and neighbours. Rescuing my little street dog, Mira, from Cyprus proved to be a godsend, as taking her out for daily walks meant that I had to leave my house and immerse myself in nature. I found myself talking to and smiling at strangers. Most days I went down to the river, just a few minutes away from my house, most days to swim. I swam in 'skins' (swimsuit only, no wetsuit) even during the winter months when the temperatures dipped below 5°C and it snowed on me as I immersed in the icy waters. Initially, I was considered a bit of an oddity, but invariably people stopped to talk to me, some of them asked to join me, and friendships began to develop. As I spent more time in the green and watery realms of nature and as I made more of an effort to connect with other human beings whilst we were all in the midst of global disconnection, something in me began to settle and an even deeper sense of inner safety began to form.

At the heart of it we are all connected. We are all one. Maybe, at the heart of it, our deepest sense of safety comes from our connection with others and with the world around us – nature. I've always believed that being in nature has many psychological benefits, and scientists are beginning to find solid evidence that being in nature has a profound impact on our brains and our behaviour, helping us to reduce anxiety, brooding, and stress, and increase our attention capacity, creativity, and our ability to connect with other people. 'People have been discussing their profound experiences in nature for the last several hundred years – from Thoreau to John Muir to many other writers,' says researcher David Strayer, of the University of Utah. 'Now we are seeing changes in the brain and changes in the body that suggest we are physically and mentally more healthy when we are interacting with nature.'

In Japan and now increasingly in the West, the practice of *Shinrin-yoku,* or forest bathing, is practised by many people who are looking to nature for restoration and healing. The term *Shinrin-yoku* was coined by the Japanese Ministry of Agriculture, Forestry and Fisheries in 1982 and is defined as making contact with and taking in the atmosphere of the forest. Rigorous scientific studies have shown conclusively that forest environments have a measurable impact on our physiology – cortisol levels are lowered along with pulse rate and blood pressure. But can immersing ourselves in nature actually affect our nervous system? These studies also showed increased switching on of the parasympathetic nervous system and dampening down of the sympathetic nervous system. In other words, being in nature makes us feel safe.

But do nature and studying the behaviour of trees have something to teach us about feeling safe? I believe they do. In the next section of my book, we leave the world of neuroscience and delve into the world of nature and trees.

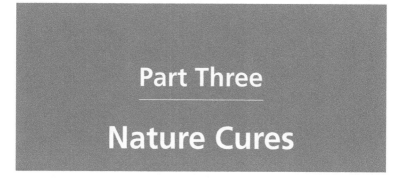

Part Three

Nature Cures

'You and the tree in your backyard come from a common ancestor. A billion and a half years ago, the two of you parted ways but even now, after an immense journey in separate directions, that tree and you still share a quarter of your genes.'
—Richard Powers, *The Overstory*

'Finland is officially the world's happiest country. It is also officially 75 per cent forest. I believe these facts are related.'
—Matt Haig, Instagram, 26 November 2019

'In the woods we return to reason and faith.'
—Ralph Waldo Emerson, *Nature*

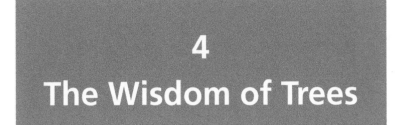

4
The Wisdom of Trees

'Trees are like people. They stress but they are beautiful when they're happy. The golden rule that I got from the storm is that you've got to copy nature and run with her and you'll succeed.'
—Tony Kirkham, Head of Arboretum,
Kew Gardens, London, United Kingdom

You might be wondering why, in a book about learning how to feel safe, I'm now writing about trees . . .

I believe that trees have a great deal to teach us about feeling safe, or rather, they remind us how to feel safe.

Have you ever been to a yoga class and stood in Tree pose? Maybe the teacher told you to plant your feet, to really spread them on the ground so you can stand strong without wobbling or falling over. Maybe they talked about grounding or earthing yourself, or to imagine putting down roots.

Have you ever sought solace in the presence of trees?

In the toughest moments of my life, and especially my childhood, I have derived comfort from being around trees – admiring them, climbing them, hugging them, talking to them, breathing in their beauty. In Guyana I grew up climbing my mother's mango, jamoon and guava trees, often despite her admonishments that I'd make the fruit go sour (apparently an old Guyanese superstition about girls who'd reached puberty climbing trees).

I am not alone in feeling comforted and steadied by being around trees.

Laura's Story

During the pandemic, I worked with Laura (38), a mother of two young children who often found herself becoming stressed and overwhelmed. Not only was she home schooling but she also worked at a demanding PR agency as well as caring for an elderly parent. She told me: 'My refuge from everything is spending time in the woods while walking my dog. I look at the trees, feel their solidity and I gather myself up again.'

Many of us experience profound feelings of groundedness and safety when we are in the presence of nature and, in particular, trees. I wonder why? Maybe they are the epitome of what it means to be strong and resilient, to withstand harsh and stressful conditions. To survive, to be safe, trees have learnt to be resourceful and to fight for their lives.

On every continent on the planet, you can find ancient life forms that have been living for thousands and even millions of years. Many of these are trees, the most elderly of which have been around for between 2000 and 5000 years, providing food and shelter for the earliest human civilizations. Man and trees have always had a symbiotic relationship – we rely on them for the air that we breathe, they filter the air keeping it clean and fresh, they provide us with medicines, food, wood, shelter, soil integrity, and they reduce our stress and anxiety levels. Man's dependence on trees – and our connection to them – is undeniable and endless but, shortsightedly, we take this relationship for granted.

So many of us these days are turning to nature to rebalance ourselves. Maybe we've got to a point when the noise and demand created by our world of technology is too much; we become overwhelmed and seek refuge in the green. I find myself wondering about the nature of our connection with Mother Nature and, in particular, trees. Maybe our connection is more physiological than we think.

Magnificent Brainforests

In his book *Trees of the Brain, Roots of the Mind*, Giorgio Ascoli, a professor at the US George Mason University describes the human brain as a brainforest in which the nerve cells of the brain, when they are enlarged a thousandfold, look exactly like trees. Similarly, small areas of the nervous system, when magnified, resemble gigantic, magnificent forests. Ascoli draws a fascinating link with how we have evolved as arboreal primates who are naturally and literally – in our neural circuits – hard-wired to love trees and forests! When I came across his work, I laughed to myself; maybe the tree-hugging hippies of the sixties were right all along and we just needed our cynical, evidence-loving logical minds to catch up.

Imagine a tree with its strong, sturdy trunk. This tree is deeply rooted, and her root plate is dense and solid, keeping her windfirm and safe. She is growing exactly where she needs to grow and there is a constant silent dialogue between her and nature around her that enables her to thrive and grow. When storms, with their heavy rains and winds, hit she bends and flexes but remains standing. She loses branches and her trunk might lean and crack but she keeps going. Even when she is lying on the ground, she sends her roots into the soil to seek nourishment, to survive and maybe even thrive.

Now imagine our nervous system starting in the brain with its central trunk and emergent nerve fibres travelling around the body, innervating and serving every cell, tissue, and muscle. How well has this nervous system been nourished and strengthened? Are these nerves strong and well myelinated or spindly, with tenuous connections and absence of myelin? Myelin is the fatty substance that surrounds the fibre axes of the nerves, protecting and insulating them and enabling them to transmit information to different parts of the body efficiently and quickly. A well-myelinated nervous system makes us resilient, able to withstand life's buffeting without breaking or falling; we are adaptable and responsive to changes in our external world because we have this deep, anchoring, and rooting safety system.

Dr Suzanne Simard, Professor of Forest Ecology at British Columbia University and author of *Finding the Mother Tree*, believes there is a physiological explanation to the unburdening sensation we experience through nature. Numerous other studies have shown that spending time in nature, in forests and with trees, has measurable physiological and psychological benefits. It lowers our blood pressure, boosts our immune system, and increases production of feel-good hormones such as oxytocin and serotonin.

Does it seem far-fetched to you that we are neurologically designed like trees or that trees can show us how to feel safe? Don't worry if it does, but the fact remains that we do refer to trees a great deal in our representations of our human selves. For example, we commonly refer to the 'family tree' as a way of describing our ancestry, where we've come from. Similarly, the term 'tree of life' which describes our universal connection to Mother Earth and our dependence on her to survive and flourish. Trees have long been associated with wisdom and knowledge; the Buddha meditated under the *bodhi* tree and achieved enlightenment from it.

In India, sadhus, religious ascetics, have always retreated to the forests for wisdom and in traditional Indian mythology, trees in their previous lives were great philosophers.

Whatever your beliefs might be, there's no doubt that we derive something both steadying and nourishing when in the presence of trees and forests, a connection that is both ancient and, at the same, grounded and rooted in the present moment. Trees make us feel safe.

The Tree of Safety

The more I considered my relationship with trees – that 'unburdening sensation' – and that of others' relationships with trees, the more I became convinced that trees can mirror something back to us about feeling safe. Maybe they can remind us about something that we, in our crazy go-harder, do-more society, have lost touch with – our innate nature. One day, while on a walk with my dog, I stood gazing at one of my favourite trees – a somewhat battered horse chestnut. Vandals had chosen to spray paint blue expletives on her trunk but she still looked the picture of joy. Her upper branches jubilantly spread outwards as if dancing – in fact, I call her Dancing Tree because of the sinuous shape of her trunk and outstretched arm-branches. She seems so resilient, so all-embracing. She feels to me to be the epitome of feeling safe despite what has happened in her life. This is when the idea of the Tree of Safety came to me (see Figure 4.1).

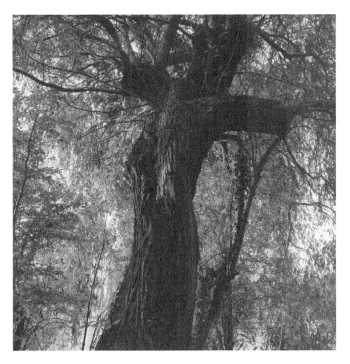

Figure 4.1 The Dancing Tree.

I am now going to introduce you to my Tree of Safety model which I believe describes our relationship with life and our ability to feel safe. A tree has three main parts – the roots, the trunk, and the crown. How do they relate to our ability to feel safe?

The roots relate to where we have come from, our history and genealogy. If we think of ourselves as being like a tree rooted to the ground, the roots of the tree and the root plate represent how grounded and steady we are, how stable we are. They are related to our ancestry, those who came before us and their relationship with the world and feeling safe. Like the roots of a tree, our roots can go deep and way back in time as well as spreading wide.

The trunk represents our life passages and stages of growth from the time of our birth until the moment we die. The annual rings of a tree reveal the tree's age as well as what it went through as it grew and even the weather conditions at the time of growth. In my Tree of Safety model (see Figure 4.2), the phases and seasons of our life are represented by the trunk of the tree.

The crown of the tree – the upper branches, leaves, buds, blossom, and fruit – is who and what we present to the world, what we bring forth – our fruitfulness, if you like.

THE TREE OF SAFETY

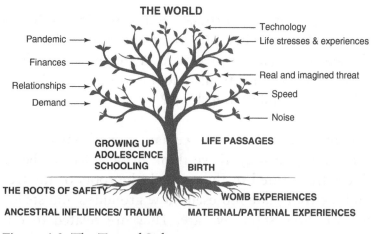

Figure 4.2 The Tree of Safety.

The Roots of the Tree of Safety

The earliest beginnings of our relationship with feeling safe come from our deepest roots – I see these as our ancestral beginnings – where our forefathers came from and their relationship with life and safety. How rooted were they? How safe were they? How safe were they materially, emotionally, mentally, physically, and spiritually? This is what creates some of your deepest roots of safety. As I have mentioned previously, epigenetics is the field of biology in which traits, behaviours, and psychological patterns are passed down through generations in our genes.

And so it is that our very relationship with life and our ability to thrive – safe or not safe – can be transmitted through our ancestry. Later, I invite you to explore your roots and, most importantly, heal those safety roots that are weakened and frayed so you can live your life more fully and joyfully than perhaps your ancestors did. I think you deserve that, don't you?

Conception, in utero, and birth experience represent the start of your journey in this lifetime. You travel up the Tree of Safety through your ancestral roots to your early beginnings, transit in your mother's womb and birth experience. There are cultures who believe that the moment of your conception plays a significant part in who you are and how you relate to life. In certain cultures, the moment of conception is considered to be a significant and holy experience. It is thought to have a significant influence on the way you make your way through life thereafter. The state of health of each parent – physical, mental, emotional, and spiritual – at the moment of conception, plays its part in the health of the soon-to-be-created gamete. Their union is seen as a coming together of energies that creates the next layer of safety for your rooting system.

There is now a great deal of evidence that a mother's experiences as she carried the foetus in her womb – the *in utero* experience – play a significant role in determining the health of her baby. Her health and nutritional status, stress levels, and environmental factors all affect the transfer of nutrients across the placenta. Research shows that it isn't just the placental exchange that is key but also the imprints on the mother's genes that affect the subsequent health of the child.[1]

The birth experience is another important aspect of your safety system. How did you come into life? Was it effortless or difficult? My mother loves to tell me that I 'couldn't wait to get out' as I was born on a hospital trolley as the nurses were wheeling my mother into the delivery room. I came with a speed which seemed to set the tone for subsequent years as I was a restless baby and this restlessness continued into my adulthood until I learned how to ground myself and be still. My mother

[1]Gluckman, P.D. et al. (2008). Effect of in utero and early-life conditions on adult health and disease. *New England Journal of Medicine* 359: 61–73.

had conceived me while she was still in grief from the miscarriage of my brother who she had carried to seven months. Incredibly, it was at a postnatal check-up that they discovered that she was pregnant with me. I sometimes wonder whether the feelings of lack of belonging that I sometimes experience are related to the unusual circumstances of my conception.

'The body remembers. There's a part of the brain that literally creates a file cabinet of experiences' says Colorado-based somatic therapist Dr Annie Brook. She has spent many decades helping people – from newborns to adults – to reset behaviours that she believes originated at birth, or even before it, through a process she calls 'persona birth journey integration'. Her work was once thought to be leading edge but she has now been joined by a growing group of experts – both alternative practitioners and Western medicine specialists – who believe that what happens before and during birth can have a lasting psychological impact.

The Trunk of the Tree of Safety – Life Passages

The initial seven years of a child's life are vital to the establishment of safety within the nervous system. When a child is first born, it doesn't know how to make itself safe, having come from the protection of the mother's womb. The primary carer of the child, usually the mother, shelters, protects, and makes the child feel safe, much like the mother tree in the forest.

When I read Peter Wohlleben's book, *The Hidden Life of Trees*, I was entranced to learn about 'tree schools' and how trees support themselves and manage to maintain stability and strength in harsh environmental conditions. He describes how 'the process of learning stability is triggered by painful micro-tears that occur when the trees bend way over in the wind' and how the tree adapts and strengthens its support system. I also read with fascination how a 'mighty mother tree' provides support to other trees but when this tree dies or is cut down the surrounding trees lose their support or, as Wohlleben describes, 'find themselves wobbling on their own two feet – or rather, on their own root systems'. Apparently, it can take 3 to 10 years before they stand firm once again after the loss of the mother tree. In this time, they have to strengthen their trunks, roots, and watering systems and become used to being exposed to more light.

> '*The thickness and stability of a trunk, therefore, build up as the tree responds to a series of aches and pains. In a natural forest, this little game can be repeated many times over the lifetime of a tree.*'
>
> —Peter Wohlleben, *The Hidden Life of Trees*

It appears that the mother tree provides the stable base for the surrounding trees mirroring the process of co-regulation that I described earlier. When she is no longer there, the other trees have to self-regulate and maybe even go through a process of dysregulation until they find their 'own two feet'.

John Bowlby, the eminent British psychologist, psychiatrist, and pioneer in the field of Attachment Theory describes in his book *A Secure Base* the importance of the parent–child bonds and how when these bonds are strong, secure, and stable, the child grows up with the ability to form healthy attachments in later relationships. Importantly, he debunked a then popular notion of unhealthy dependence between baby and mother, saying that babies come into the world biologically wired to form attachments and that this is necessary for their survival in the world. In other words, our secure base in the world, our ability to feel safe in the world, is created from our earliest beginnings when we are handed into our mother's arms at the time of birth and begin our journey of co-regulation – learning how to feel safe in the world from the secure base of her protection.

But we cannot remain forever tied to our mother's apron strings and, at some point, we need to cut loose and start to find our own safety. This is where we start to self-regulate or stand on our own trunk, sorry, two feet. This can show up like the 'terrible twos' as the toddler starts to establish their place in the world, their authority. They explore and stretch the boundaries and, while this can be challenging for parents, it is a necessary and healthy part of the individuation process. The little human being is starting to feel safe to be who they are – 'This is me!' they are saying when they have their toddler tantrums.

Gail Sheehy is the US journalist and sociologist and author of 17 books, including the highly acclaimed

Passages, which helped millions navigate their lives from early adulthood to middle age.

'With each passage of human growth, we must shed a protective structure. We are left exposed and vulnerable – but also yeasty and embryonic again, capable of stretching in ways we hadn't known before.'

—Gail Sheehy, *Passages*

Research shows that adverse childhood experiences affect the degree of myelination of the nerve fibres in the brain and body. In other words, growing up in an environment that is unsafe and traumatic affects the development of the nervous system. But it goes beyond this. Let's think about that tree again and the seed or cutting that it came from. Was that cutting strong and healthy? Did it have strong roots and internal water and nourishment systems to enable optimal growth? Or was it spindly and malnourished? Childhood trauma affects our very own rooting and growth systems so development and optimal growth is challenging.[2]

The Crown of the Tree of Safety

I would like you to consider the following questions again because how you present yourself in your world

---

[2]Sanders, M. et al. (2018). Trauma-informed care in the newborn intensive care unit: promoting safety, security and connectedness. *Journal of Perinatology* 38: 3–10.

represents the crown of your safety tree. This is your 'overstory':

* Who are you today?
* How do you show up in the world?
* How well do you inhabit your skin?
* Are you thriving or surviving?

In a forest, the overstory is the uppermost layer of foliage in the forest, it forms the canopy. It is how you show up in the world. As I've said before, I've worked with so many people who appear to be doing well, their 'overstory' looks good – foliage strong and vibrant – and then the signs of *dis-ease* appear and they might even topple. They become ill, sleepless, lacking confidence, unhappy, and sometimes for no obvious reason, unable to cope, unable to stop, burnt out, addicted, depressed and hopeless, and more.

We can be so caught up in our overstories, the content of our lives, that we don't realize that healing needs to be done – until we fall over. Hopefully, we embark on a journey of understanding and healing our weakened and damaged roots.

To withstand life's buffeting, we need strong roots and trunk. External stress comes from all directions and we need deep strength and stability to withstand external forces of life, to be able to lean in. The work begins, to go back and repair and heal the damaged roots – I call this the Real Work.

The Real Work

I introduced the idea of 'the Real Work' in my second book *Fast Asleep, Wide Awake*, where I invited my readers to go deeper, to discover the true source of their sleep problems. It takes courage – and energy – to do the Real Work. This is no sugar-coated, saccharinized spiritual journey. We need powerful resources to do such work and I will help you if you're ready to take this path. Doing the Real Work of finding inner safety means not being afraid to cry, or ask for help, or step into the unknown – a void that can feel unsettling and even frightening. But it also means no longer living a numbed-out, anaesthetized life and being able to feel such joy – such as you've probably never known before. It means being able to thrive.

Doing the Real Work of feeling safe often means going back and discovering who you really are. This could mean going back and exploring your roots and where you have come from as well as making sense of your life experiences and how you are presenting yourself in the world – your roots, your trunk, and your crown.

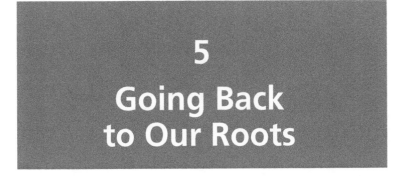

5

Going Back
to Our Roots

'Maybe you are searching among the branches, for what only appears in the roots.'

—Rumi

Have you ever watched the BBC television programme *Who Do You Think You Are?* The popular programme, in which celebrities trace their family trees, started in 2004 and is still going strong. Millions of people watch the programme. We seem to be fascinated to understand where we come from because it helps us to understand who we are and why we are who we are. Many people are also undergoing ancestral DNA tests in an attempt to understand who they are and where they have come from. Looking back and joining the dots – discovering one's family tree – helps us to find our place in the present reality and strengthens our sense of belonging. It also helps us to understand our relationship with feeling safe.

Early Beginnings

Our ancestors and their relationship with safety, our parents' life experiences, the womb experience, the birth experience, the first seven years, schooling, who you hung out with (or didn't). These are the roots of your relationship with safety. And how? There is now an abundance of evidence that shows that stresses, strains, and traumas are handed down through generations in our DNA. Trauma can leave a chemical mark on genes that is transmitted down through our lineage; to feel safe or not safe in our world can reside within our genes.

As a sleep expert, I have come across this in my work in cases where people turn up to see me for help with their sleep problems. Solving sleep problems is sometimes a little like detective work – we sleep the way we live, the way we eat, move, breathe, drink, think, and relate to other human beings. I'm renowned for saying 'Live well, love well, sleep well'. I usually start with many questions trying to piece together the jigsaw puzzle of who this person is, their lifestyle, what they are going through in their life, discovering the root of why they can't sleep. In some cases, I can't find an obvious pattern or reason why they're not sleeping so I might go back further to find out more about their ancestry, their parents. I call this Autobiographical Enquiry. By completing this enquiry, I'm finding out more about their roots, what has made this person who they are? Are their issues deeply rooted in the traumas of those who came before them? Are they now responding to life – feeling safe or not safe – from events that have happened in the past?

Sarah's Story

I worked with 29-year-old Sarah who had been signed off from her workplace for more than three months. She was suffering from panic attacks and extreme anxiety – and she couldn't sleep. She said she had always been this way since childhood – sensitive, anxious, and sleepless. Talking to her it was clear to me that she had inherited something that was playing out in her current life. I asked about her parents and their lives. She told me that her mother's mother, her grandmother, had died suddenly of cancer when Sarah's mother was 15 years old. Sarah's mother was forced to leave school to become the family breadwinner and care for her younger siblings. Her mother had always carried the mark of the sudden and traumatic loss of her own mother along with a deep sadness and regret that she hadn't had the opportunity to continue her education and follow her dreams of becoming a nurse or doctor. Sarah said her mother often half-jokingly referred to herself as being 'thick' and 'uneducated'.

Fast forward to the current day and I saw how this was played out in Sarah's life as she described classic traits of her own 'imposter syndrome'. She was bright and intelligent and clearly respected and

(Continued)

valued at work, but constantly felt 'not good enough' walking around with a constant fear of 'being found out'. She said other people thought of her as 'ditzy' and a bit silly, not very bright. She carried the fear of failure to bed with her, finding it hard to let go and relax. She told me she was even afraid to close her eyes at night and woke up every night with nightmares. Sadly, she had found that cigarettes, alcohol, and a weekend recreational coke habit took the edge off her fear and anxiety. I saw clearly why she was on a very slippery slope and I really wanted to help her.

Later in the Resources section of my book, we will return to Sarah's story and I will explain how I worked with Sarah and the astonishing results we achieved.

In my work I have met many people like Sarah who have ended up in a bad place but there's no obvious reason why this has happened. What might bring them to me is a pattern of perfectionism and overwork that leads to burnout and insomnia but these are the overstory. What is underneath it? Does something lie in their roots that has brought them to this place, to me?

On an energetic level, traumas are inherited 'even if the person who suffered the original trauma has died, even if his or her story lies submerged in years of silence,' says family therapist Mark Wolynn.[1] 'Fragments of life experience, memory, and body sensation can live on, as if reaching out from the past to find resolution in the minds and bodies of those living in the present.'

Wolynn says that the firstborn daughter, in particular, is likely to carry what her mother hasn't resolved. A descendant could be atoning for an ancestor's misdeeds without realizing. His words make me think of my sister who did not survive our childhood and the traumas that had carried through our ancestry; her roots were weakened so that when the lupus attacked her system, she had nothing to fight back with. I also reflect on Sarah's journey and how for years she had thought of herself as 'thick and ditzy' until she began healing the trauma pattern related to her mother's unfinished schooling.

Weakened Roots

Inherited trauma can remain stuck in the familial body for generations until it is healed. Or rather, until it is time for it to be healed.

My friend and gifted body worker, Chris Sritharan says: 'We can only heal if there is a surplus of resources' and this makes me wonder if generational trauma shows up for healing at exactly the right time. By this I mean, I wonder whether there comes a point in our family

---

[1]Mark Wolynn (2016). *It Didn't Start with You: How Inherited Family Trauma Shapes Who We Are and How to End the Cycle.* Penguin.

history when there is someone who has the resources to heal weakened roots and so, in their lives, they have to face a 'topple' (shortly, you will understand exactly why I am using that word) which provides the opportunity for healing and not only for them, but for the whole family line and, in particular, those who are yet to come.

Your ability to feel safe today could be influenced by your relatives who came before you and their relationship with life. As human beings we are an extremely resilient species, surviving wars, disasters (both natural and man-made), traumatic insults in our own lives, and more recently, the stresses wrought by the Covid-19 pandemic – and yet we keep going. Bessel van der Kolk in his book, *The Body Keeps the Score*[2] described how stress and trauma become stuck in the body and, until they are released, we cannot fully thrive. We live defended, rigid lives, holding ourselves tight in a state of armour against imagined threat.

> 'Traumatic experiences do leave traces, whether on a large scale (on our histories and cultures) or close to home, on our families, with dark secrets being imperceptibly passed down through generations. They also leave traces on our minds and emotions, on our capacity for joy and intimacy, and even on our biology and immune systems.'
>
> —Bessel van der Kolk, *The Body Keeps the Score*

[2]Bessel van der Kolk (2014). *The Body Keeps the Score*. Penguin.

This armouring can be passed down through genera-tions, affecting our ability to feel safe and to live whole and fulfilling lives.

In the process of healing my own relationship with feel-ing safe, I went back through my history and learnt more about my roots and my ancestors. This was when I began to heal profoundly . . . and finally I could sleep. In my work, I have been privileged to be able to help many people embark on a journey of healing their own weak-ened roots. It is a journey . . . and not one that can be completed overnight.

Mala's Story

The first time I met Mala (34), a teacher, I was drawn to her sweet nature. I felt there was a true innocence about her – almost childlike at times. She had a good life – very happily married and in a job that she was good at and enjoyed. She and her hus-band were thinking about starting a family – they were settled and ready. But in January 2017 – four months after they were married – she started hav-ing sleep problems. She saw her doctor and various sleep specialists and was prescribed sleeping tablets which made her feel 'terrible' so she stopped taking them. She had heard about my work and eventually came to see me after a few years of struggling to sleep and trying various strategies. To her, her sleep problems had come completely out of the blue and

(Continued)

she could see no reason why they had suddenly started. I too could see no reason why in her every-day happy life the insomnia would suddenly appear. As usual, we covered the obvious – daily routines, lifestyle habits, work stress – and there was nothing obvious there. Next, we embarked on her Auto-biographical Enquiry.

I discovered that at the age of four Mala had been sent to three different care homes. Her parents were from India. Her mother was schizophrenic, and her father was an alcoholic, so living with her parents was not deemed to be safe for Mala and her two siblings. She had a much older sister who was sent to live with an aunt and Mala and her older brother were sent to foster homes. At the time of seeing me Mala didn't know if her father was alive but her mother was now more stable and somewhat inde-pendent although still needing a lot of support.

Her story saddened me and I was keen to explore several practical strategies for Mala to try out first before we went any deeper. As I anticipated, there was no real change to her sleep, which confirmed my suspicion that the root cause of her sleepless-ness lay deeper within. So, at her second session we talked about her childhood and I gently introduced the idea that her sleep problems might be related to her earlier traumatic upbringing. She told me she felt shocked but also 'relieved'. She had been told by specialists to challenge her beliefs and had embarked on Cognitive Behavioural Therapy (CBT) programmes but they'd had no effect at all. Only left her feeling as if she wasn't trying hard enough.

Can you see how the formative years of your life – the early trunk experiences – can lead to deep weakenings, Peter Wohlleben's 'painful micro-tears' which show up in later life? And why at this point in Mala's lifetime? Years later, when Mala was able to make sense of her story, she made the connection that it was when she was thinking about starting her family, something that she and her husband were so excited to do, that the insomnia had started. In her words: 'I've often wondered whether, subconsciously, married life and the thought of having a family triggered something in me given my own traumatic childhood experiences.'

But I'm jumping the gun. Let's go back to Mala's story.

Mala's Story

In our second session, not only did I introduce the notion of childhood trauma but I also told Mala that I felt I wasn't the right person to work with her. I strongly felt she needed the right kind of therapy to address the trauma that was stuck in her

(Continued)

body. I could see and feel her frustration – she was desperate for help. I took her through several breathing techniques and *chi kung* exercises which she could use at night to help her to relax but deep down I knew she needed to do the Real Work. I recommended healing modalities such as Craniosacral Therapy and Psychotherapy with a particular leaning towards healing trauma in the body. I sent her away, hoping that she'd have the courage and faith to explore this avenue and asked her to stay in touch with me. A year later Mala wrote to me. She was reading *The Body Keeps the Score* and had, as I had recommended, done powerful healing work. She had been 'sleeping like a log since'. Not only did she work on her sleep but she also realized how, for most of her life, her self-esteem had been very low. She had suffered panic attacks but never really did anything about them.

Mala wrote to me again while I was working on this book. She said: 'I'm still doing the healing work and I regularly take time out to focus on my breathing. I'm better at shutting down my self-critic. I take more pleasure in nature and go for long walks ... taking time to be in the present and enjoy small things rather than rushing to get it over with.' She now has a one-year-old daughter and is expecting her second child.

We cannot think our way into feeling safe (and sleeping deeply) if at the heart of it we are still carrying the wounds of our childhood – much as we would like to. This is why CBT couldn't work for Mala and for many of my clients who come to me with sleep or stress-related problems. The part of the brain that is trying to help us to survive, the limbic system, lies deep below our rational brain and it is not very good at pretending or denying. In fact, I often say that when we're in survival mode we're not using our 'front brain', or neo-cortex, the part of the brain that is relatively recently evolved and helps us to think and process information logically and rationally. Instead, we're using our 'fear brain', the deep, primitive limbic system. So the healing has to go deeper and back to our roots and beginnings. Mala has suffered severe uprootings and although she had managed, in many ways, to thrive, it was only when she was ready to confront and heal her early childhood experiences and where she had come from, that she could begin to feel truly safe.

Where Do You Belong?

Belonging plays an important part in our ability to feel safe. Our sense of belonging comes from our rootedness – where are roots are planted and how strong and deep they grow. Consider your answers to these two questions before reading on:

- Where do you feel you truly belong?
- Where is home for you?

In the same way that plants need the right soil and conditions to grow, so do human beings. We need to feel a sense of belonging to feel safe, to survive. According to Abraham Maslow's Hierarchy of Needs there are five categories of needs for people to survive, of which belonging is a key one for optimal living. Have a think about it for a few seconds – imagine yourself walking into a roomful of people at a party. As soon as you walk in you sense the vibe in the room. If you paid attention to it, you would notice a feeling in your body – usually your gut – that tells you; 'I belong here' or 'I don't belong here'. You reach for a drink – you're at a party after all – but many people reach for a drink because their body has registered a feeling of 'I don't quite belong here (yet) and I need something to help me relax'.

The question of 'Where do I belong?' is a potent one when considering your relationship with feeling safe. Suta Guy Rawson, a coach and therapist, says that for him the place where he belongs is 'the setting in which I can truly thrive and give of my unique essence'. Where is this place? Where is it for you?

When I think about my own roots, I can see that there were so many uprootings and transplantings; moving from one place to another. Maybe this is why I'm not the best traveler, taking a while to settle down and ground myself into my new environment no matter how comfortable it might be. Maybe this is why I have a terrible sense of direction and have been very lost several times when I've been away from my home. Such as the story

I shared with you in the prologue of this book about my terrifying and transformational ordeal in the Portuguese mountains.

It took me a while to understand that my apparent poor sense of direction which, by the way, has improved significantly since getting to the root (excuse the pun) of the problem, and difficulty settling in strange environments was because of my weakened roots of belonging. These have resulted in me feeling dissociated and unsafe when away from home.

This may be the case for you too and perhaps you can think about your own roots as I tell you about mine.

My Ancestral Story

Late eighteenth century – Great-grandparents left India (Uttar Pradesh or Calcutta? Poor records so it is unclear) to emigrate to Guyana, South America, to work as indentured slaves in the rice and sugar cane plantations.

The Guyanese culture is a strange one; the poor relation of the Caribbean, this is no picture-postcard Caribbean island, with golden sand beaches and turquoise sea. The coastal strip of Guyana is brown and muddy because the waters of the Amazon River drain through the rainforests here and flow out to

(Continued)

107

sea. Many people think of the Jonestown massacre of the 1970s in which Jim Jones, the American psychopathic leader of a cult, took his following into the Guyanese rainforests and then fed them Kool-Aid laced with cyanide. More than 909 people were murdered. Other people might know Guyana as the ex-colonial country in South America that has the highest single-drop waterfall in the world – the Kaiteur Falls. Or, they may recognize it from the BBC documentary *The Land of the Lost Jaguar* – for Guyana's wildlife is breathtakingly beautiful and relatively untouched.

My grandparents and parents were born in Guyana. My mother's family in particular were poverty-stricken, with nine of them living in a single room in a mud hut.

Being transplanted to another soil in this way resulted in the loss of some spiritual and cultural stability anchors – a significant source of safety. My ancestors were Hindus but many of them had to abandon their faith and religion to gain employment. As I grew up, it was common to hear stories of wife beatings, incest, alcoholism, cousins who died from drinking poison or hanging themselves.

Both of my parents spoke of the harshness of their upbringing – the beatings at home, the punishments at school – my mother still bears the scars of a particularly savage beating dealt to her by her own older brother. Theirs was not a safe or gentle upbringing and survival was paramount. My father had grown up with extreme violence as my paternal grandfather was an evil man, driven by a strange mix of desire to succeed, tenacity, and alcoholism. My paternal grandfather was driven and ambitious and he managed to work his way out of indenture and eventually bought the land and factory his family had toiled on for decades. So, in relative terms, Dad's family were relatively wealthy; they even owned the village bus, Susheela.

1961 – My parents left Guyana for England, traveling for 30 days on the Estania ship. My mother was heartbroken to leave her beloved mother and sisters to whom she was very close but Dad was hell-bent on self-improvement and had his heart set on becoming a doctor, lawyer, or engineer. Again, life in this foreign soil was hard. Racism was rife in the 1960s in South London and Mum worked hard all day in a factory packing boxes to put my father through college.

My sister, brother, and I were born in London and my father eventually graduated with a degree in engineering. However, perhaps because of the racial situation in England at the time, my father was

(Continued)

unable to find work that fulfilled him and utilized his skills as an engineer and he decided it was time for another uprooting.

1972 – My family and I returned to Guyana on BOAC (British Overseas Airways Corporation) Airlines in the hope that job prospects and quality of life might be better.

1970s – Racial unrest between the two main ruling parties in Guyana headed by the Indians (the People's Progressive Party or PPP) and the blacks (the People's National Congress or PNC). Secondary school children were being forced to spend a year in the army doing national service before they could continue their schooling. Reports of rape and abuse of Indian schoolgirls by black soldiers during their term of service were common.

1978 – My sister and I were forced to return to England to live with a family in Croydon. A financial arrangement was set up by my father and the head of the family who unwillingly took us in so we could continue our schooling in England.

My sister and I found ourselves in an all-girls school filled with middle-class white girls who looked at me as if I was a complete oddity. And I was. I spoke differently, looked different, and, I was told, smelt different. I retreated completely into my shell and hardly spoke and in my school reports teachers used words like 'self-effacing' and 'reticent' (both of which I had to look up in the dictionary) to describe me. I missed running around with bare feet, chasing the dogs, climbing trees.

During this time my father stayed in Guyana and continued, with ferocious drive and energy, to grow his business. At the peak of his career, he had an engineering company employing more than 30 people and his work gained recognition and kudos. His company designed and built the country's first floating bridge that stretched across the Demerara River; a treetop walkway in the rainforests; a world-class cricket stadium in Georgetown, Guyana's capital; the first athletics stadium; and an Olympic-sized swimming pool. My father was a perfectionistic high achiever for sure. He continued to strive hard throughout his life and even had a meeting with his general manager the day before he died while lying in intensive care in hospital. He was made a Fellow of the Royal Society of Engineers in 2005 but still he remained a tortured soul.

Can you see the patterns of not-belonging and not-your-home? These uprootings and transplantations can cause weakened roots, unstable moorings – lack of safety.

Maybe this is why my father's moods could be violent, unpredictable, and frightening to all of us – my siblings, my mother, and me.

Maybe this is why my mother was always sickly, needy, and unwell.

Maybe this is why my sister died suddenly, traumatically, at the age of 42.

Maybe this is why I, for so many years, faced so many mental and emotional challenges and struggled to find safety for so long, before I succeeded.

Maybe that's why I've written this book.

Different Types of Roots

My story is not pretty, but I share it so that you can understand how our roots, our earliest beginnings, lay the foundations for who we are later in life. When I tell my story, I visualize in my mind's eye various roots – some of which are strong and deep and thriving. For example, the roots of my ambition and drive that have enabled me to become successful, to achieve academically, to gain recognition for my work; I believe these are strong and thick. They travel deeply through the soil back to my ancestors who were driven to leave their homeland, to toil hard once they arrived in Guyana, to overcome adversity and buy their freedom back. I attribute much of my success to being connected to these particular roots. I don't think of myself as particularly driven or ambitious but because I'm so connected to these 'achievement' roots it sometimes feels as if I have no choice but to strive and succeed. For a time, striving was all I did. But I wasn't thriving because my roots were weak and damaged and so I was unable to feel joy, a sense of belonging and safety. It affected my relationships and friendships, and fear and loneliness dominated my life. My healing came – and these roots were healed – when striving no longer worked and I became ill. My breakdown/breakthrough forced me to revisit these roots of striving and to find the safety that now allows me to live from a different place – one of abundance and thriving.

There have been other losses and abandonments, but my story is not about being a victim. I have other roots too and it was by discovering and strengthening these roots that I now find myself in the place of feeling deeply safe – and safe enough to write this book. These roots are joyful, playful, and creative. They bring forth my love of dance, books, and nature. They connect me with the Divine and help me to rise up and see the interconnectedness of life. They give me my faith and courage and they constantly help me to find true meaning and healing in adversity: never giving up hope.

The Tree That Toppled

How do we start to bring healing to these weakened roots? Where do we even begin to heal the trauma that our ancestors suffered that was passed down through the lineage and that is now showing up in our everyday lives? Is this even possible?

The Turner Oak Tree

I found the story of the Turner Oak profoundly moving. Here was a story that illustrated to me everything I believed about life, how it can tear us up from our moorings and how we can rediscover solid ground and our grounding roots of safety.

In October 1987, there was a storm of unprecedented strength and unpredictable winds in the United Kingdom. I was 23 years old and visiting my parents' home in Croydon, south of London. Miraculously, I slept through the storm but was unable to go to college the next day because several trees had been blown over, blocking roads and train tracks so transport ground to a halt. I didn't know this at the time, but Kew Gardens, home to more than 14 000 trees of incredible diversity and beauty, took a hard hit in that storm. More than 700 trees toppled and were uprooted. The Turner Oak was violently uprooted, her entire root plate torn out of the soil. She lay forlornly on her side in the gardens. She was more than 200 years old and the oldest and biggest tree in Kew Gardens. The staff were devastated. Apparently, she had been unhealthy before the uprooting and while some of the botanists wondered if this might be an opportunity to save her, a last chance if you like, most of them believed she would die and have to be chopped up and removed from the grounds.

They hoisted the Turner and propped her up, planning to deal with all of the other fallen trees first and then come back to her last. It took them three years to eventually return to her and when they did, they got a big and wonderful surprise . . .

The Turner Oak was thriving! In fact, she was a picture of health! Her roots had re-established themselves and were feeding her foliage abundantly. Since the hurricane she had put more than a third of her growth back on. Her branches are strong and sturdy and her foliage vibrant and verdant.

And why?

It is a myth that the roots of a tree grow deep. They are in fact held in a shallow root plate much like the base of a wine glass. Over the years, and before the storm, the footfall around her and on top of her root plate had been relentless. People walking around her had compacted the soil, which had lost its porosity and aeration, and simply, the roots of the Turner couldn't breathe or drink. They had become weakened and undernourished and, thus, vulnerable when the storm hit.

The story doesn't only end well for the Turner Oak. The story of nature picking her up and shaking her roots out heralded the beginning of a new era in tree management in gardens across the world today. Over the years, companies have developed machinery specifically for aerating the soil around tree plates, so-called 'air cultivation'.

Years later when I heard this story, it touched me deeply. My own life with its shocks and uprootings and picking myself back up and growing stronger. All of the people I have worked with over the years – including those who I worked with at the psychiatric clinic – who had been through the most challenging circumstances and eventually come to see that what they experienced was not a breakdown but a breakthrough, painful as it felt at the time. Life can wear us down, it can press down on us so hard that we feel we can't breathe and sometimes we fall over and the falling over comes in the form of the losses, the big illnesses, unexpected shocks that tear us out of our moorings, leaving us feeling we'll never know how to get back up again. But we do. I have done. We find our feet-roots again and we reground and we grow stronger. As a result of the toppling over and uprooting, we are safer and can thrive.

But not everyone does. It takes courage and a hell of a lot of energy to get back up but this is the real work of life. This is the only way we can grow.

What did the Turner Oak story show me?

We have to keep our soil aerated. We all need to breathe deeply and we need the freedom and space to do this. Life can compact our soil, pressing down on us, so we become smaller, weaker versions of ourselves. We're stuck and just surviving.

We need the right nourishment to thrive, to reach our full growth potential. This might mean that we need to seek new, more fertile soils. We need to be uprooted.

Once transplanted, we need to heal and strengthen our roots so we can thrive in richer soil. But first we must go back and reclaim, rediscover our roots – then the healing can begin.

When we are nourished deeply from our roots,
we can't help but grow
into who we are meant to be.
We can't help but bear the fruit
we are meant to bear.
This is God – or nature – given,
depending on your beliefs.
Unavoidable.

Part Four

Doing the Real Work (of Finding Inner Safety)

Practices and Resources

> 'I look at my family's ancestry the same way I look at the roots of a plant. Both go deeply into the earth, fed by the nutrients of time until the roots are strong enough to support the great fruitfulness.'
> —Tiffany McDaniel, *Betty, an Autobiography*

Getting Ready to Do the Work – Before You Get Going

> 'The tools come before the work.'
> —Jackie Boothe (therapist and healer)

Doing the Real Work (of Finding Inner Safety)

'We are what we repeatedly do.'

—Aristotle

It is time for me to share with you the tools I have been practising myself and sharing with my clients for more than 25 years. Are they mere 'tools'? I struggled with using this word as it felt devaluing, given their potential to effect deep and life-changing transformation. Some of them I have developed myself, by a process of trial and error, and many are based on ancient practices and traditions that have been around for a very long time. However, for simplicity, I am going to use the word 'tools'.

But before we start, I want to share a few key messages about using these tools:

1. **Tools are only tools until you use them.** Sounds obvious but how many times have you signed up for a course and didn't apply the learnings, or bought a piece of equipment and didn't use it? Gym memberships are the ultimate rusty and expensive tool!
2. When used regularly, tools become '**practices**'. As we deepen into practice, it becomes a way of life, an embodied experience, and perhaps something we don't need to think about because it has morphed into our way of being. For example, think about the way that you take a shower or bath or clean your teeth. Hopefully, unless you're a teenager (!), you don't have to think too hard about whether you want to practise good hygiene or not; it's second nature and you make time for it without too much effort because you know

120

that it is important for your wellbeing to feel clean. I want to reassure you that practising these tools will enable them to become second nature when used regularly as you start to notice and feel the benefits.

3. This is when our practices become 'resources'. We become resourceful or rather, we are resourced to deal with life, to face its challenges, and do the work on it (see Figure P4.1).

TOOLS ⟶ PRACTICES ⟶ RESOURCES ⟶ RESOURCEFULNESS

Figure P4.1 The journey to becoming resourceful.

4. **Support** – The work of finding inner safety can be trial and error. Ask for the right help and, trust me, you will find it. Who you ask depends on your personal belief system. Having faith helps. You might pray for guidance to your God, your Higher Self, your ancestors, the angels or fairies. Or you might ask your friends – preferably the ones who you feel embody that sense of grounded safety that you are seeking for yourself. Tell them what you are practising and enlist their support to help you do the work. Journalling can also help this process.

Explore the tools that I'm offering you. Apply them and make them your own and you will start to experience your own Aha! moments.

5. **Intention** – Create an intention for how you want to feel. Intention-setting is powerful. This is your vision of where you want to be and how you want to feel in the future. It enables you to make choices in the NOW

moment to get to where you want to be in the FUTURE. You choose differently and with awareness. How do you want to feel? I'm sure you want to feel safe, but how does that feel to you? Can you find your words? Preferably words that are positive and not based on what you *don't want to feel*.

Send the *right* words into your subconscious rather than the *wrong* words to create a powerful vision of how you want to feel. What I mean by this is that sometimes people say 'I don't want to feel X, Y or Z', but how *do* you want to feel? The problem with identifying how you *don't* want to feel, important as this might be, is that you can end up programming exactly what you don't want into your subconscious mind. For example,

*Right now, **don't** think of pink elephants. Whatever you do, absolutely don't think of pink elephants.*

What are you now thinking of?

Marauding, huge pink elephants, right? The way our mind works is that it does tend to fixate on and embed the most powerful words we use so if you say 'I don't want to feel afraid', the most powerful word in this sentence is AFRAID.

Think about what feeling safe means to you, how it would feel in your body. Go back to moments when you have felt safe – maybe you were stroking your pet or listening to your favourite music while cooking a nice meal, or hugging someone you love. You might find it helpful to go back to the word clouds at the beginning of the book and find your words and write them down.

Create your Feel Safe vision and aim for it.
6. **Readiness** – Are you ready to do the work? Have you reached a point of acceptance of where you are right now – toppled over, burnt out, hope-less, joy-less, or feeling unsafe? Or maybe things aren't really so bad but you want them to be better. You want to feel more joy, to know what it feels like to truly thrive. Readiness is key. It will spur you to action and keep the fire of transformation burning.

In my first book, *Tired But Wired*, I describe an ARC of transformation in which we can take the measure of our readiness for change. In my model we first of all become **Aware** of our role in creating whatever change we want to have happen in our lives. We stand at the centre of our lives taking full **Responsibility** for ourselves and the **Choices** we now need to make.

Awareness
Responsibility
Choices

Now we know that we are not victims of our circumstances, we don't have to be defined by our past, we can choose differently and thus live different lives.

I wrote my first book in which I described the ARC in 2010 – more than a decade ago. At the time, I have to confess that I perhaps saw life in a more linear way – if I do this, then I'll get that . . .

The journey isn't a linear one. I knew this then but I *really* know it now. In fact, the journey probably looks a bit more like Figure P4.2.

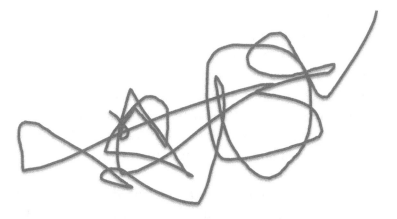

Figure P4.2 The chaotic spiritual journey.

If you examine this apparently chaotic visual more closely, you will see that it is actually composed of a series of mini-arcs. The journey of doing the work of finding inner safety is up and down and round and about. But eventually, we get to stages when we realize that it is time to stand at the centre of our lives and take responsibility, choose differently. Along the way, we have our Aha! moments, our awakenings and realizations as we melt away the layers of armour that we've built up around ourselves over the years – **de-armouring** until we get to our centre from which true safety emanates.

7. Finally, before we really get going . . . **the work isn't done until we're done.** There isn't an end point as such, although we do get to feel safer and safer as we practise. Sometimes, life starts to throw at us bigger challenges and curve balls but by then, we are deeply

and non-negotiably resourced. We ride out the storms, eventually getting to the other side and enjoying the calm while it lasts.

So we find the tools, we practise diligently while holding the intention for where we want to go, and in doing so we build our resources and become resourceful and steady in ourselves, even during life's storms. *This* is the journey to finding true safety.

Practices and Resources Index

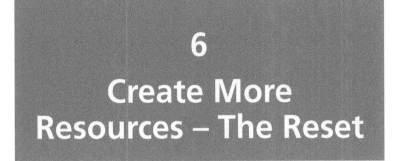

6
Create More
Resources – The Reset

'The journey of a thousand miles begins with a single step.'
—Lao Tzu

Taking the first steps towards inner safety might require you to gather your resources. If you think about the story of the Turner Oak, the gathering of resources is the equivalent of the arborists propping the tree up, putting supports in place around her so she was upright. At the time, they didn't realize they were giving the mighty oak the opportunity to start her healing journey. What I will share with you in this section is the equivalent of propping yourself up so you can start your healing journey too.

Can you remember, as I said earlier, that you need a surplus of resources to embark on the journey of doing the Real Work? It takes energy to create the momentum to make different choices and create new habits. It takes energy to face the demons we might encounter on the path to finding inner safety. Healing takes energy.

How do you go about getting this? Years ago, I realized that, even though I'm a sleep expert and this is what I do – I help people to sleep – what I actually do is resource people so they are able to heal.

What Are Your Energy Levels Right Now?

Can you give yourself a score out of 10? Zero is exhausted and completely burnt out so I'm hoping you won't go there. Ten is amazing energy, fully resourced.

Take a note of your energy levels – I know this isn't terribly scientific, but it is a quick and useful way of monitoring your resource level. To get stuck into the Real Work, you need to be feeling at least a 6 or 7.

What I am now going to share with you are key practices for getting you resourced so you can embark on the journey of finding real inner safety. The problem with many other toolkits which are purely cognitive or psychology based is that they begin with the Real Work. This is hard to do if you don't have energy, if you're not sleeping, if you're struggling to survive. Going through the reset will help you to find more energy so you can do the work with more ease and grace. It's the equivalent of filling your car with petrol before you embark on your long journey.

Press the Reset Button

Many years ago I discovered that I was doing something incredibly simple to help my clients to break out of their patterns of burnout and insomnia. I took this simple method, and it became known as my 5 Non-Negotiables (5NNs) that I went on to write about in my books and talk about in my presentations. I have to describe them again here because I also realized that the 5NNs are what also help to break patterns of survival. It can help to bring about the shift from living from the sympathetic nervous system – triggered and activated – to the para-sympathetic nervous system of safety and thriving.

When I think about the story of the Turner Oak, going through the reset is the equivalent of propping the tree up and putting supports in place to enable the journey to feeling safe to begin. This is where it starts.

When we're running in survival mode, we can lose sight of who we are, the things that make us feel joyful, confident, and happy. We forget our childhood dreams and passions. We become dried out and dispirited. Survival energy makes us run on fear. We feel choiceless. We feel unsafe.

Alex's Story

I worked with 42-year-old Alex, a highly intelligent ex-professional rugby player who is now practising law. For months he hadn't been sleeping well. Waking in the early hours, unable to get back to sleep, worrying about everything. Eventually, he'd give up and just start working. When we met online, I could see he was running on 'fizzy' survival energy. He hardly made eye contact and I could tell that he was not-so-surreptitiously looking at his phone and emails throughout the session, anxious about work he felt he needed to be doing rather than being on our call.

There was a lot going on with Alex – he hinted at past traumas and talked about suffering from 'internalised Tourette's syndrome'. He also admitted that he'd been thinking suicidal thoughts and about self-harming – a strategy he had resorted to in the past when he hadn't felt great. At this stage, I wasn't sure if medical intervention was needed but we agreed to make some small changes and see what happened. He agreed to keep in touch with me and let me know if he felt he needed medical help.

Less than 24 hours later Alex wrote to me to say that he couldn't believe how different he was feeling. All we'd done was to get some nourishment into his roots.

And how?

- He cut back coffee – he had been having two strong cups to start his day and more throughout the day.
- He started eating breakfast.
- After our call he started drinking more water.
- He started prioritizing and valuing his sleep.
- That night he put his laptop and phone away earlier and went to bed earlier – with an old-fashioned book.
- He didn't take his phone with him.
- He didn't look at the time when he woke during the night.
- He didn't look at the phone as soon as he woke up in the morning.
- He went out for a run at lunchtime.

This might sound a bit basic, but the thing is, the body needs the basics. It needs the right nourishment, the right treatment to function in the way it is meant to. Our nervous system needs the right treatment otherwise it gets nervous and we think we're under attack.

I was surprised at how quickly Alex responded but he had once been a professional athlete so maybe his physiology was primed.

At our next session less than two weeks later, I was even more pleasantly surprised. He even looked different;

the first time I'd seen him he looked grey and slightly unfriendly, refusing to make eye contact. Now he was talking animatedly, his eyes were shining, and he had a broad grin on his face! He was feeling happier at work and was finding time for his passion – writing and practising standup comedy, something he'd nurtured a longstanding passion for!

What had happened in such a short space of time?

Alex had definitely 'fast tracked' my method but his case is not unusual. I see changes usually within a week if my clients are really committed to doing the work to get the right nourishment down into the roots. Often they start off feeling a tad cynical – how can such small changes make such a big difference when they're feeling so bad?

Imagine a neglected plant – maybe a pot of parsley – sitting on the windowsill. You've been so busy and caught up with life and you've been forgetting to water the plant. It is looking half dead and wilting. Guiltily you get your watering can out and give the poor parched plant what it needs. Within minutes you start to see a difference in the plant. It starts to stand upright and it even looks greener. You can see life in it again! This is what happens when we get the first drops of nourishment into our soil. This is what happened to Alex.

Getting Started

Here's where you get started on building your resources. These tools are based on my 5 Non-Negotiables[1] methodology and you want to aim to practise for 7 to 10 days. I promise you – you will notice the change. If you want more details on this aspect of my methodology, I recommend that you read my second book, *Fast Asleep Wide Awake*, where I explain the protocol in more detail.

The following will help you to get started on cleaning up your energy:

1. **Eat within 30-45 minutes of rising.** How do you feel when you wake up? Are you mentally already fast-forwarding into your day? Are you waking up with

---

[1] Where does the term 'the 5 Non-Negotiables' come from? Many years ago I was running a stress management workshop for a group of traders at a well-known investment bank in Canary Wharf. It was an awful session. I was at the start of my speaking career so I didn't have anything near the confidence I have today. It was 7 p.m. and there were more than 50 people in the room. The bank had laid on refreshments for them, including beer and wine. They were raucous and ill-behaved and I was struggling to do my job. When we got to the toolkit section of the programme, in desperation, I yelled (to make myself heard) 'I'm going to share five things that will improve your relationship with sleep and your energy and then I'm going to get the hell out of here! I don't actually give a s**t whether or not you do them but if you, I know they will make a massive difference!' Thus the 5 Non-Negotiables were birthed!

a sick, anxious feeling in the pit of your stomach? These are all indications that you are running in survival mode. Eating breakfast enables you to make the shift from sympathetic nervous system/fight or flight to the parasympathetic nervous system/safety and thriving. Include a source of protein in this breaking of fast. Avoid intermittent fasting or similar diets if you are running in survival mode.

2. **Avoid caffeine.** Don't use caffeine as a substitute for food, ideally drink no more than two cups of tea or coffee per day and avoid caffeine after 3 p.m.

3. **Hydrate.** Aim to drink at least two litres of water a day. Alkalize the water by adding a pinch of natural sea salt and a squeeze of lemon.

4. **Prioritize rest and sleep.** Get to bed earlier – around 9.30 or 10 p.m. – and read a book, journal or meditate to calm your nervous system. Don't oversleep. Don't obsessively check the time at night.

5. **Create an electronic sundown.** An hour before you get into bed, start to withdraw from technology. Leave your electronic devices out of the bedroom and avoid looking at them when you wake during the night (which is entirely normal). Give yourself at least 20 minutes before you look at your mobile phone in the morning.

6. **Move.** Get moving to get your energy levels up and to shift the low mood. Brisk walking is good too. You don't need to spend hours in a gym. The key is to change your energy state in the morning even if – and especially if – you haven't slept well. My favourite

movement if I haven't slept well is to put my favourite music track on and to either dance, skip, or hula hoop for at least five minutes to shake off the inertia.
7. **Avoid the news and social media.** Especially first thing in the morning and last thing at night. Start your day feeling hopeful and end the day feeling trusting.

As I've said, this methodology is described in much more detail in my previous books if you want to learn more. For now, I'm inviting you to really commit to this journey, much as part of you might be feeling some resistance such as:

I can never eat breakfast in the morning – it makes me feel sick/I don't have time.
I have to have my coffee first thing in order to function.
I hate drinking water.
I can't go to bed that early.
What?! Get my phone out of my bedroom? Are you mad?!
I'm so tired . . . I can't possibly exercise.
Any other............ (Feel free to fill in the blanks)

I remind you that I've been doing this work for more than 25 years – longer if you include my own journey – and I've heard (and used) every excuse. My methodology has even worked with patients in the psychiatric clinic where I worked. Trust me, this clean-up is essential and once your energy levels have lifted (we're aiming for at least 6 or 7), you're ready to go deep. You are resourced.

Feel Resourced – What to Expect

Once you've committed to your reset practice (approximately 7 to 10 days for most, even less for some – remember Alex's story?) you will start to feel

- more energized, even if you haven't slept particularly well;
- more optimistic and hopeful in general, even if things aren't going well;
- less obsessed with how you are or aren't sleeping;
- more able to delve into the real source of your unhappiness, insomnia, or burnout;
- ready to explore your relationship with feeling safe.

What you have done is to put the right nutrients into the soil. You're finally nourishing your roots so they can begin to thrive. Now it is time to aerate the soil.

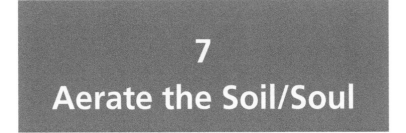

7
Aerate the Soil/Soul

'There is one way of breathing that is shameful and constricted. Then, there's another way: a breath of love that takes you all the way to infinity.'

—Rumi

Like the soil around the root plate of the Turner Oak, we too can become compacted and restricted by life. Unable to breathe, unable to thrive. Once the Turner Oak had her supports in place, finally her roots were able to breathe and thrive. Similarly, in my work and personal journey, I have noticed that breathing – aerating your soil – plays a key role in the journey to safety. So much so that when I accidentally wrote in my notes 'aerating the *soul*' I decided that I needed to use this word, as this was exactly what I had personally experienced as well as witnessed with countless clients and patients when they started paying attention to their breathing.

In this section of the book, I am going to explain how and why breathing can bring about immense transformation, as well as sharing simple practices to get you going.

Compacted Breathing

Years ago, I noticed how many of the people who were coming through my health screening laboratory in London's Square Mile were breathing suboptimally. Their companies had sent them for their health assessments and, as I said right at the beginning of the book, my lab tests showed they were running in survival mode. Sitting for long hours compacted their breathing; caffeine and adrenaline sent the breath up into the chest even more, leaning into screens. Their fast lives left them unable to take a deep breath. Ironically, at the time, I didn't realize that I was also living a compacted life and couldn't breathe. My restricted breathing wasn't because I was working flat out but because of the traumas of my childhood that had left me in state of constantly holding my breath as if waiting for something bad to happen.

When we don't or can't breathe fully, we start to feel restricted and restrained, stuck in unconscious tramline patterns of behaviour that might not be serving us. We hold in our feelings of pain and hurt – they stay trapped in the body, eventually causing illness or chronic exhaustion. (Don't forget, this is the 'freeze, don't move' state.) Past hurts, if not healed and released, stay stuck in the body, in our very cells. They become our way of being. They feed our addictions and neuroses. They occupy our cellular spaces, leaving no room for hope, joy, and love. In other words, they stop us thriving.

This is how compacted-ness shows up in the human psyche.

Learn How to Breathe

I met 39-year-old Jessie Laute down by the river near my home. I was doing my usual wild swimming and I didn't even notice her watching my friend and me as we, giggling, shivered uncontrollably trying to get dressed after a cold autumn swim in the River Thames. She came bounding up to me with a broad smile on her face and asked if she could join us one day. Naturally I agreed as we're always on the lookout for fellow crazy wild swimmers. Now Jessie and I have become friends and, as well as having the occasional dip together, we've really got to know each other. It turns out that she is a gifted breathwork teacher who has been running a successful practice teaching people how to breathe for years. As we got to know each other, a beautiful friendship began to emerge and I was touched by her story.

Jessie Laute's Story

Thirty-nine-year-old Jessie was born in the UK to Indian parents who were born in Africa. She had a very successful career in human resources in various high-flying City firms, enjoying the financial rewards, the busy sociable lifestyle, and travelling around the world. It was while working for a prestigious bank in the City, where she'd been headhunted, that her life started to spiral out of control. Two weeks into the job, she realized that things

(Continued)

143

weren't right, it wasn't the right job for her. But she kept going for two years. During this time, she wasn't taking care of herself, and her health deteriorated drastically. She was drinking to cope with the stress, eating badly, not exercising, and not sleeping. Her personal relationships started to suffer and then, of course, her work. The classic burnout spiral.

Realizing that something needed to change, she left and headed off to Brazil to work for a social enterprise company. It was here that she started to 'breathe out and let go'. She hadn't realized how long she'd been holding her breath. She began to have fun – genuine fun – exploring her passions and values and finding out what she really cared about, which included working with people. She decided to train as a coach and it was during this training that she attended a breathing workshop. It changed her life. She connected with a sense of stillness and peace that she'd never before experienced. She continued going to the classes and each time she found herself opening up and releasing tears and emotions that she didn't even realize were there. The next revelations came when she started uncovering deeper insights into difficult events that had happened in her past – and making sense of them and letting them go.

The biggest insight came when she uncovered the trauma she'd experienced when her father died tragically when she was 16. There had been a big fire in her family home. Jessie, her three siblings, and her mother had escaped unharmed, but her father died in the fire. She was carrying so much guilt and shame in her body, on a cellular level. Consciously she knew that it hadn't been her fault but subconsciously, and on a cellular level, her body was still holding on to the experience even though it was 20 years ago. This began Jessie's journey of healing the trauma of her father's death.

As I have said previously, the body keeps the score. When Jessie started allowing herself to breathe, she discovered that trauma had shaped her life in ways that weren't good for her, she was only surviving.

Like the toppling over and uprooting of the majestic Turner Oak, her breakdown-breakthrough had allowed vital aeration of her soul and now she could start to thrive.

Jessie continued practising breathwork to heal her father's death and it was during one of these sessions that her father came to her in a vision and said 'this is the start of your spiritual journey'. This was an awakening that led her to start meditating and exploring other energy healing modalities. She started running her breathwork consultancy and now goes into many corporate environments teaching groups of people how to get out of their heads, get back into their bodies, feel what needs to be felt, and release stored emotions that are blocking their ability to thrive – in a safe way.

Jessie's journey is ongoing. As she said in our interview 'life still happens' but the trauma is no longer defining her life and choices. She now knows that her strength lies in allowing herself to feel what she needs to feel and, as a result, she is now able to help so many others. She had 'never felt safe enough to put down roots but now I do'. Relationships with family members have been difficult as her siblings have struggled themselves to come to terms with their father's death but Jessie continues to find safety and peace in her breathing practice.

Take a Deep Breath

Breathing deeply aerates our soil. It aerates our soul. After an uprooting or breakdown, we create space in our life, or rather, we are forced into new and unaccustomed space and we have to stop. And then what? Now we have room to breathe.

Learning to Breathe

I learned how to breathe after I returned from my awakening in Australia in 1999. I found myself at the *Sivananda* Yoga Centre in Putney doing an introductory yoga course. I was hooked after the first session. I had done yoga before but now, unlike the past when I would leave the class before the end just when everyone was lying down to breathe and relax ('I don't have time for this relaxation rubbish!'), I would stay and allow myself to lie there in *savasana* or corpse pose, trying to surrender, trying to let go and relax. It was hard. Decades of holding myself tight made it impossible for me to be still.

Fast forward more than 20 years and we all know about breathing now. In fact it is probably the latest wellbeing craze – breathwork workshops, Wim Hof breathing, holotropic breathing, SOMA breathwork, circular breathing, kundalini breathwork, Buteyko breathing. I think there is a global realization that we need to learn how to slow down and take a deep breath.

Learning how to breathe was a revelation to me. And to my clients too. So many of them came to me with their stresses, worries, and insomnia. I simply showed them how to breathe . . . and then I watched the transformation.

You would think that something that we do twenty to twenty-five thousand times a day should be so easy, so natural. But it isn't. We get into patterns of holding our breath thinking we're holding out pain when really we're holding it in. We think we are bracing ourselves against life, keeping ourselves safe from (usually) imagined threats when what we're really doing is making ourselves feel more unsafe.

When we don't breathe fully, we don't inhabit our bodies fully. We become dissociated and numb. At some point in our lives we may have learnt that this was a helpful thing to do, that it would stop us feeling a pain or trauma at that time that we didn't have the resources to deal with. Maybe we were young so learning how to not feel, to block out (in) uncomfortable feelings was preferable to feeling them.

Returning to Sarah's Story

We had a breakthrough the first time I encouraged Sarah to breathe. She had been through her 'clean-up' and was sleeping much better most nights but was still anxious. I noticed that in our sessions she had a tendency to lean forward on the edge of her sofa. We were working together online but still, her anxiety was palpable. I asked her if she felt she could lean back against the sofa and relax and she replied that she felt she really couldn't. It seemed to make her feel uncomfortable. Sitting in this way meant that her posture was curled inwards, her solar plexus blocked off, armouring herself against imagined threat. She said that she felt she had to lean in otherwise she might miss what I was saying to her, might 'get it wrong'. So I suggested that she sit as she was and simply close her eyes and notice her breathing. I asked her to focus on one exhalation and explore whether she could make it longer. At this point she

---

sat back and sighed. After less than a minute of noticing her breathing, tears began rolling down her cheeks. 'Why am I crying?' she asked.

We will return to Sarah's story again.

Becoming acquainted with your breathing is a profound and rewarding journey and it can start right now. One breath at a time. Are you ready? You might choose to join a breathwork class or even try a personal session with a practitioner (please see the Further Resources section). To get you started, I introduce you to a couple of simple and gentle practices that you can work into your daily routine immediately. Starting a breathwork practice doesn't have to entail sitting in lotus position for hours or even attending a class. You can start right here, right now.

Practice 1: Notice the Breath

Notice Your Breathing

What is it doing right now? Don't try to change it, simply allow it to do what it has been doing all along until you paid attention to it.

Have you been holding your breath while reading or listening to my words?

Are your shoulders tight?
And what about your jaw?
Have you been gripping it?
Is your breathing deep?
Do you feel it in your belly or does it feel stuck in your chest, shallow and tight?

Go Deeper

If you find that your breathing is shallow and restricted in your chest, lie down comfortably. Don't get into bed if you might be in danger of falling asleep! Using blankets and cushions, make yourself comfortable and warm.

Notice your breathing. Place your left hand on your chest and over your heart. Place your right hand on your belly.

Allow your breathing to settle and deepen, feeling the weight of your hands on your body. Can you allow your breath to reach deeper into your belly?

Start to gently prolong your exhalation but don't force it. Imagine you are breathing roots out through your lower body – belly, hips, legs, and feet.

Don't worry about your exhalation – it will take care of itself. Simply, gently making the exhalations longer OOOOUUUUUUTTTTTTT as if you are breathing roots out through your feet and deep into the earth.

Send those roots deep down into the earth.

As you breathe out your roots of safety, repeat to yourself:

IT IS SAFE FOR ME TO BREATHE.

IT IS SAFE FOR ME TO BREATHE DEEPLY.

I AM SAFE.

I AM SAFE IN MY BODY.

I AM SAFE IN MY LIFE.

Practice 2: Take 5 a Day/Morning Practice

This simple practice is one that I do most days. On days that I don't I might find myself rushing around, feeling ungrounded and even overwhelmed with everything I feel I have to do.

When you wake in the morning, avoid rushing to open your eyes. With your eyes closed, simply check in with your breathing. What is it doing right now?

Simply follow five exhalations. Doing this might make you want to breathe in a different way – your breath might deepen so you feel your belly expand. Alternatively, let it do whatever it wants to do. Simply follow it.

As you notice your breathing, ask yourself 'How am I feeling right now?'

Just a simple check-in to start your day.

It would be good if you could repeat this exercise as you go about your day. Perhaps find three other times when you simply notice five exhalations at three other times in the day. Maybe before you have your lunch or while you make a cup of tea. And then, last thing in the day when you turn your light out, follow five exhalations to help you to slide effortlessly into velvety sleep.

This simple practice helps you to become acquainted with yourself and how you are feeling rather than being constantly caught up in the mental realm – always thinking, often over-thinking.

Breathe.

Come back into your body.

Come back to yourself.

Practice 3: Sigh it Out

This is a really effective practice for letting go of emotions or stuck energy as you go about your day. We tend to sigh spontaneously as we go about our day but if we bring intention to our sighing it becomes a powerful therapeutic practice in its own right.

Mira Sighs with Relief

To remind you, Mira is my rescue dog from Cyprus. She came to live with me in 2020 during the Covid-19 pandemic and, to be honest, I'm not sure who was rescuing whom. When she arrived, she was terrified and every noise I made startled her; she'd had a traumatic life on the streets of Cyprus so it's not surprising that she felt unsafe. However, over time, as her trust in me grew, she started to feel safer and more settled knowing that her life with me was now her 'forever home'.

I love it when she comes to sit next to me, resting her head on my lap. I stroke her beautiful fox brown coat and she sighs with contentment. It happens every time and my daughter now calls it Mira's 'fufff'. As she fufffs, I can feel her settling and softening into relaxation. She has decompressed.

When we sigh, it drops us into feelings of calm and contentment. Try it right now. Take a big, exaggerated breath in, hold it in for a second or two and then sigh it out through your mouth. Make a sound as you do so. Make a sound of relief as you sigh.

Try this again, this time exaggerating the exhalation and making it longer.

Imagine sending this exaggerated sigh out of the soles of your feet, as if you are breathing out roots, so this prolonged out-breath makes you feel safe, grounded, and connected to the earth.

Notice if you start to feel softening anywhere in your body. Maybe your shoulders drop and relax, or your eyes and jaw soften.

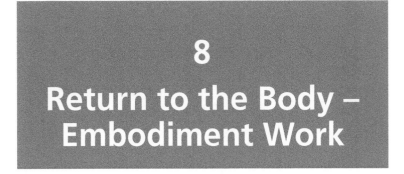

8
Return to the Body – Embodiment Work

'In order to change, people need to become aware of their sensations and the way that their bodies interact with the world around them. Physical self-awareness is the first step in releasing the tyranny of the past.'
—Bessel A. van der Kolk

Breathing is the bridge that takes you into the body. When Sarah started to gently explore her breathing, it took her into the feelings and emotions that had become trapped in her body. She asked 'Why am I crying?' but I encouraged her to not judge the tears but simply to allow them. So quickly we can end up making judgements and arriving at conclusions that aren't helpful. We get caught up in stories about why we're feeling a certain way – which might not even be true – and in the process we get stuck in the mental realm of thinking and processing and not actually allowing ourselves to properly feel what needs to be felt. This is one way in which emotions become stuck in the body. It is so easy to be distracted – an uncomfortable wave of emotion arrives and we pick up our phones and throw our attention into social media or some other electronic distraction. An hour of scrolling passes in the blink of an eye and the wave has passed. Or has it? Often it hasn't – it remains trapped in our cells and tissues just waiting for us to be still, maybe in bed at night, and then it hits us again.

Does this resonate with you?

Feeling safe isn't only about challenging your thoughts or changing your stories or ways of communicating with yourself and others. It is also about the freedom and liberation of your body. Our bodies are often held so tightly because of the pressures we face out there, they become internalized into the pressures we hold in here which affects everything – our neck, shoulders and jaw, our cardiovascular system, our energy levels, our digestion, our sleep, and more.

If we could just learn how to feel what needs to be felt rather than freezing, numbing out, checking out, leaving our bodies, dissociating, seeking to control everything out there, seeking perfection – whatever our favourite pattern tends to be.

As we learn to feel we may encounter layers of frustration, worry, irritation, and impatience. If we allow ourselves to bravely go deeper we might even encounter guilt, anger, rage, shame, loneliness, and sadness – all of the things that we feel in our humanness. But as the poet Kahlil Gibran writes, 'Your joy is your sorrow unmasked' – in order to get to the sweet kernel of joy and happiness, we have to learn to sit with uncomfortable feelings and feel them. But how do we do this?

I have spent decades working on this, doing various workshops, training programmes, attending conferences, and reading books but thankfully, you don't have to. It can be so hard to feel what needs to be felt – years of conditioning that have taught you to numb out, shut down, not feel, stay busy. Life is filled with distractions that offer easy escape from unpleasant feelings. But remember, the rewards are amazing – peace, contentment and happiness, more energy, deeper connections with other human beings. Have I convinced you that this work is worth doing?

I really hope so. I'm going to offer you a few simple but profound somatic practices for getting back into your body. I remind you, the word 'somatic' comes from *soma* meaning 'of the body'. Here we return to the concept of 'interoception' that I introduced you to earlier – the body's ability to perceive the sensations and what is happening within. The more you work on your interoceptive abilities, the more you can become attuned to your bodily responses in certain situations. You might notice that around certain people or in certain environments your jaw clenches or your heart rate speeds up. The more you pay attention to the sensations in your body, the greater you become at meeting its needs. The need for comfort or support or the need to leave a situation or speak up. The need to not watch the third episode on catch-up TV or scroll endlessly on Instagram but to pay attention to your tiredness, switch off, and go to bed and get a good rest.

By the way, this is not a self-indulgent journey. The more you pay attention to your body, so you become a better friend or parent or manager as you start to notice more about what is happening in the environment around you.

What follows are body-based practices for you to use as you go about your day. They are a vital part of your healing toolkit as you journey towards finding inner safety.

Practice 1: Notice Your Body Awareness

Simply take a moment to notice your body and how you are holding it:

- Are you sitting, standing, or lying?
- How are you holding your head, your neck, your shoulders, your back, your legs?
- Notice the levels of tension in your body.
- Can you feel any tension in your face, your chest, your back, your legs, your belly or stomach?
- Is your jaw clenched or relaxed?
- Are your hands gripping?
- Are there any places in your body where you feel ease?
- Any places that feel tight?
- Can you feel your heart beating?
- Is it racing or does following a steady, regular pace?

- Can you even feel it?
- Does noticing your body create any tension or anxiety for you?
- How are your energy levels right now?
- Do you feel energized and maybe even eager or impatient to get going or do you feel lethargic, sluggish, and tired?

Too often people ignore their bodies' whispers and needs so they end up, at the end of the day, dehydrated or eating and drinking the wrong things.

Where are you physically right now? By this, I mean what does your body feel like and what is it trying to tell you? What needs is it trying to express right now?

Maybe as a result of paying attention you now want to move to get more comfortable – lean back or lie down. Maybe you want to roll your shoulders down and back to release some tension. Maybe you want to open your mouth wide and release the tension in your jaw. Maybe you want to go and get something to eat or drink.

Body awareness is such an important part of this healing journey.

Practice 2: Locate Your Trigger Points

The aim of this practice is to become aware of how your body responds to stress. How does it let you know you've become triggered or activated? Think of a recent time when you felt triggered – the more recent the better:

- How does your body tend to respond?
- Where do you tend to hold the stress in your body?
- What are your trigger points?
- Do you know?

For many people, stress is held in their shoulders, chest, stomach, and belly. It is often held in their face, in the space between the eyebrow and in the jaw and this tension travels down into the neck. Breathing becomes constricted and shallow, which exacerbates feelings of un-safety. These are your body's physiological red flags. Your body is asking you to pay attention.

For me, emotions such as anger, fear, worry, and sadness tend to lodge in my stomach, around my solar plexus. I start feeling nauseous and it affects my breathing. If it goes on for too long, I start to feel tired and low. My body droops and wants to go into hiding. This is one of my well-worn patterns and I now know how to work with it. But the first step, as I've said previously, is awareness. Get to know your patterns and then they don't take over and cause dis-ease in your mind and body.

If you haven't been able to spot your patterns, simply pay attention for the next few days. You don't need any major upsets and traumas to start noticing your body responses to stress. Simply pay attention – when you're driving and you end up stuck in traffic, or standing in a queue in a supermarket and someone is taking forever with their payment and discount vouchers – notice the impatience, feel how your body is responding, what is your breathing doing?

The next step is to see if you can gently encourage your body to regulate itself. Can you shift your attention to your feet, feeling your feet on the ground or if you're sitting in traffic by scrunching and relaxing your toes, or hunching your shoulders and relaxing them? Another release could come from taking a breath in through your nose and exhaling in a prolonged sigh as I showed you in the previous practices.

The more adept you become at noticing your trigger patterns, the better the chance of halting the cycle of freezing and numbing emotions into your body. You become better at releasing as you go about your day. When you can tune into your body's wisdom, the next step is for you to commit to trusting it.

Practice 3: Feel Joy and Pleasure

While it is important that we work on facing and feeling unpleasant feelings, it is also good to notice the times when we feel good and to embed them even more in both our bodies and our memories. This is another way of creating safety in your body and one which we will come back to in more detail when I share with you how to rewire your brain and nervous system so it has a positive rather than a negative bias.

Remember a time and place when you felt good. It might be a place that you go to time and again and here in this place you feel relaxed, peaceful, or even joyful. It might also be with a certain person or people – when you are in their presence you feel safe and calm in your body.

Take a moment and think: who is this person or what was the place? The person might be a friend or family member or they might be someone who is now deceased but as you think about them and the role they played in your life, it brings a sense of inner peace to you. This person might be someone who is wise and reliable, whom you trust. Some people don't have a such a person, but they might bring to mind their Higher Self or an angelic being. If you can't think of a place as such then you might imagine one – a fantasy location that you saw in a film or a beach hut looking out to the sea.

Now close your eyes and think of this person or place and, as you do so, begin to notice the sensations and feelings in your body. Notice if you are breathing more deeply, if there is more relaxation in your back, in your jaw, neck, and shoulders. Notice if you are holding yourself in a different way.

Feel the calm in your body. Feel the safety in your body. Know that it is a gift you can give to yourself at any time, especially when you feel your body is tense and tight. You can choose to give yourself some ease in this moment. It doesn't mean that all of your problems are solved, it doesn't mean that everything in your life is perfect, but it does mean that you are worthy of taking a deep nurturing breath, you are worthy of comfort and ease, and you are worthy of knowing what this feels like in your body.

If you have grown up feeling the pressure to lean in to life, and spent most of your adult life leaning in, you might not even know what it feels like to feel relaxation in your body. This simple exercise can help you to learn physically how to let go.

Practice 4: Sense Your Environment

In this exercise you will use your senses to ground you and bring you into the present moment. This is a powerful way to regulate your nervous system.

Look around wherever you are and notice what you see right now:

- What can you smell right now?
- What do you notice in the air?
- What do you physically feel on your body?
- The chair underneath you, the clothes against your skin, your glasses on your face.
- Cool breeze against your skin.
- What do you notice touching your body in this moment?

- What do you hear right now?
- What sounds are in the environment around you right now?
- Maybe you can hear traffic or birds outside.

Finally, pay attention to the taste in your mouth.

- What can you taste in your mouth?
- Maybe something you ate earlier or the toothpaste or mouthwash you used. Maybe you can taste the cup of tea you just had.

As you do this exercise you can mentally and silently tell yourself what you are noticing:

- I can see . . .
- I can smell . . .
- I can feel against my skin . . .
- I can hear . . .
- I can taste . . .

When we are feeling overwhelmed or stressed, we can find safety by simply tuning in through the senses to the sensations in the body, noticing and describing these sensations in detail.

When we pay attention to what is happening in our bodies – the areas of tension and stuckness – we can start to relax and release.

The act of paying attention to what is happening in your body can sometimes seem to intensify the feeling. You might pay attention to your heart racing and feel as if it is getting worse, but by continuing to notice it and describe it (*I am noticing that my heart is beating fast*...), the act of describing and paying attention will usually bring you to a place where the spinning will stop, the racing will slow down.

Practice 5: Take a Walk in Nature

In this simple practice you take a walk in nature but take no electronics with you. Don't take your phone or music or anything that might distract you. All you are going to do is walk in nature, listen, and feel. Feel your feet on the ground as you walk. Listen to the sounds around you. Birds singing, trees rustling, the wind. If it is raining feel the moisture on your skin.

Notice if you become impatient or even bored. Notice if you crave some form of distraction or noise. How does the impatience or boredom feel in your body? Breathe in deeply, exhale all the way out to your feet, through your feet. Feel your feet on the ground. Keep coming back to the sensation of your feet on the ground. Keep coming back to the sensations in your body.

The aim is to listen, smell, breathe, and simply feel your way back into your body.

Practice 6: Jump Back into Your Body – Heel Drops

This is an exercise that I love to do when I feel I've really 'left' my body, either because my mind is racing with some sort of conflict I've encountered, or I've simply spent too much time staring at a screen. This simple but profound exercise was taught to me by the gifted Embodiment Coach and therapist, Marcela Widrig. I often invite my audiences to try this exercise during my presentations and they always love it. It can be quite energizing too so it's a good one to do if you've been sitting for too long and you need to find the motivation to get active and go to the gym or out for a run.

Please listen to your body and if you feel any pain in your joints – hips, knees, or ankles – while doing it, stop.

For extra challenge you can do this exercise with eyes closed but perhaps have a chair or table nearby for additional support, if you feel you need it:

• Stand with bare feet about hip width apart. Slightly bend your knees to bring some softness into your legs.
• Feel your feet planted firmly on the ground. Spread your toes and allow yourself to feel the heaviness of your body being supported by your legs and feet.
• Close your eyes, lift your heels, and then come up onto your toes and drop back down onto your heels.

- Allow your upper body to be really relaxed, jaw loose, shoulders loose, arms loose and dangling by your sides so when you drop down you feel like a rag doll but you are landing solidly on your feet.

Don't forget to breathe as you do this exercise (as we often do when we're concentrating). Breathing in as you come up and out as you drop down. Maybe even introducing a big exhaling sigh as your heels descend.

Practise this 8–10 times or even more if you'd like to. Coming up you're on your toes, dropping back down onto your heels, feeling your lower body heavy and grounded.

Then with eyes still closed, feel what you can feel. You should have an enhanced awareness of your lower body. It might even feel tingly or heavier.

Enjoy the feeling of getting out of your head and back into your body.

When you're ready, open your eyes and go about your day with this greater awareness of your feet and lower body.

You can even do a simple, perhaps gentler, version of this exercise if you wake up during the night finding your mind racing and can't get back to sleep. Keep your eyes open in the dark, do a few small heel drops to drop you back into your body. Nothing too energizing. When you're ready get back into bed, keeping the awareness of your feet.

Practice 7: Discover *Chi Kung* Shaking

If after doing the heel drops you still feel you need more to help your awareness to drop into your body, try introducing some shaking into the exercise:

- Still standing with feet hip width apart, feet spread and firmly planted on the ground, knees soft, eyes closed, upper body loose and relaxed.
- Bring some gentle swaying and shaking into your body while feet remain firmly planted.
- Again, don't forget to breathe as you do this exercise.

Practise this exercise for a few minutes or even longer if you wish. Trust me, it is energizing and you will feel great after you've done it. You might even want to do this with some energizing music on and allow the enjoyment of the music to guide you back into your body.

When you're done, with eyes closed, again allow yourself to feel the energy tingling around your body.

Enjoy the rooted groundedness in your lower body.

Other times, reconnecting with your body might bring you into an unexpected sense of playfulness and fun. Go with that. Be silly if you want to. This doesn't have to be hard and serious work. Another thing I love doing when I'm 'stuck' in my head and trying to either shake off some stress or find a creative solution to a problem is to get down on the floor and roll like a ball. Lying on your back, bring your knees up to your forehead and start rolling back and forth. This is also a great exercise for massaging out the spine and a perfect counterbalance to sitting hunched over a computer screen.

Practice 8: Find Comfort and Ease

You may find that when you practise some of these techniques, particularly the softer, gentler ones, some emotions arise in you. It is good to have ways of soothing and comforting yourself when doing this work and applying a simple technique based on the Havening Technique could be really helpful.

The Havening Technique was developed by the US neuroscientist Ronald Ruden as a form of trauma therapy.[1] I am offering you a simple version of his technique that can be used alongside any of the practices that I've shared in this section of *Finding Inner Safety*.

Havening Technique

- Cross your arms, place your palms on your shoulders, stroke your arms downward to your elbows, and keep repeating brushing your hands down your arms.

---

[1] Ronald Ruden (2013). *Havening, A New Way of Healing*.

- While performing this stroking action you can repeat the words:

  - I am safe.
  - I am safe in my body.
  - I am safe in my life.

And it really is as simple as that. Enjoy the feeling of being back in your amazing body. Welcome home.

Go Deeper

The practices I now share with you are aimed at taking you even deeper. If you have done the reset, you will be feeling resourced to go deeper. I remind you, the key is regular practice. The exercises I share with you, when practised regularly, can really help to steady you – and in so doing, create a sense of inner safety. In this age of instant gratification, we can become obsessed with instant results, but real knowledge and wisdom take time so be patient, keep practising, and you will reap the benefits.

You have become familiar with your breath and have learnt to return to your body, and this journey is ongoing too. Now the focus turns to drawing inwards even more and starting to befriend your inner world – the place where safety truly resides.

The nature of getting to know your inner world is very personal and not all of the practices will work for all people. Keep an open mind – try them and see what works for you. The aim is that, over time, you will have your own set of well-used resources – your own personal toolkit, if you like.

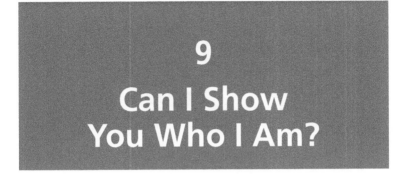

9
Can I Show
You Who I Am?

'The real gift of love is self-disclosure.'
                    —John Powell, *Why Am I Afraid to Tell*
                                        You Who I Am?

'Good, better, best. Never let it rest. 'Til your good is better and your better is best.'
                                        —St Jerome

'How many of you grind your teeth at night?'

If I ask this question of my audiences, in a room of
around 100 people, at least 10 of them will put
their hands up.

Bruxism is excessive teeth grinding or jaw clenching.
A dentist might recommend that you wear a mouth
guard if it is damaging your teeth. She might even talk to
you about stress. I talk about perfectionism.

There is nothing wrong with striving for excellence or seeking to improve your life but excessive perfectionism can come from a deep place of not feeling good enough and not feeling safe so you seek to control everything in your external world. Your inner dialogue is hard, punitive, and filled with must do's, should do's, have to do's. In fact, psychologist Dr Albert Ellis actually coined the word 'musterbation' (!) to describe the excessive drive that makes someone feel as if it's never good enough, they can never stop, they *must* try harder. Good, better, best . . .

My Story of Perfectionism

The St Jerome quote above is a poem I was made to recite every morning at school for four years when I lived in Guyana. I attended a strict Catholic convent run by nuns, and standards were high. Perfect for strict Hindu parents who really wanted their children to achieve way and beyond their own dreams.

My perfectionism drove me hard. So much so that I was afraid to speak at school for fear of saying the wrong thing and I developed a stammer so teachers wouldn't pick on me. I got to a point where I realized that I actually had so much to say but I needed to perfect my delivery. Almost overnight, I stepped into a different persona – someone who appeared to be confident and sociable. Someone who later became a public speaker, standing on stage and commanding the attention of large audiences and speaking on TV and radio.

But even this wasn't all of me. I was standing on stage and looking confident but inside I wasn't feeling great. It was only when years of healing removed layers of unhelpful conditioning that it felt safe for me to show the world who I really am and truly believe it.

It can take courage and safety to show others who we really are. To speak up in our closest relationships, to assert ourselves in our professional lives. Many of my clients grind their teeth, carry tension in their necks and shoulders, and suffer from headaches and migraines. They are often high achievers who say 'yes' to everything and everyone while saying 'no' to themselves. Until they burn out or their sleeplessness becomes unbearable.

In order to speak our truth we have to feel safe.

We have to love ourselves enough to know that our words are worthy of being spoken, heard, and received.

It goes beyond wearing a bruxism-preventing mouth guard.

This aspect of the Real Work takes time and patience. As I said before, I can offer you the tools and it is up to you to practise so they become resources and you become resource-full.

I offer you these tools from my heart. I invite you to open your heart, enjoy them, and be gentle with yourself as you use them.

As before, I recommend that you read through the exercises and choose one or two to incorporate into a daily practice for 7 to 10 days.

If any of the exercises bring up feelings of sadness, simply allow the feelings. You can also use the Havening Technique described in the previous chapter to bring you some additional comfort and soothing if necessary.

Practice 1: Identify Your Inner Perfectionist

You are going to need your journal or a notebook for this exercise.

I want you to sit comfortably, lean back, close your eyes, and feel your feet on the ground. Follow a few breaths and observe them getting deeper and dropping into your belly.

Now bring to mind a recent occasion when you told yourself you *had* to do something in a certain way or something needed to be done that only you could do. It could be something as innocuous as hanging the washing out or stacking the dishwasher but it's something that you think no one could possibly do as perfectly as you do and so it *has* to be done by you.

Or you might think of a recent occasion when you did something and you really didn't think it was good enough even if others told you it was. It might have been something you cooked or even a presentation at work. Whatever it was, it just wasn't good enough.

Find your scenario, recreate it in your mind as if it is happening right now. Where were you when it happened? What was happening around you? Re-create the scene as vividly as you can.

Now I'm going to challenge you to try to hear the voice that was telling you it has to be done by you, it has to be done exactly like this, no one else can help you, you have to do it without help.

Or try to hear the voice that said it simply isn't good enough. This is terrible. Look at them laughing at you behind your back. No one really thinks much of it or you!

Can you identify the voice? Can you hear that it isn't you? Who is it? Is it a parent or teacher from years ago at school? Don't worry if you can't identify the voice or even separate it from your own inner voice. The important thing is to open yourself up to the realization that it is not a loving you who drives you in this way. It is someone who is harsh, unkind, and even punishing – and someone who you can choose whether or not to listen to.

Can you have some fun with this? If so, I invite you to give the voice a name. I'm sharing with you now that I have a slavedriver of an inner perfectionist called Miss Trunchbull – do you know who that is? She tells me that I can't rest, it has to be done just so, I can't ask for help, and I'm not allowed to stop until my inbox in empty. It has to be perfect.

And what do I do with Miss Trunchbull when she pops up? I pause, notice her, and then I reassure her. That may sound odd but in essence, I'm reassuring a very young part of myself – little Nerina – who learnt a long time ago that she needed to do things perfectly in order to feel safe. She needed to be in control, to hold on to life tightly and not let go, she needed to keep trying harder (but it would never be good enough).

I have several Miss Trunchbulls – and you may do too. Another who says I have to exercise even though my knee is aching or I haven't slept well. Another who says I look fat/unattractive/not as good as everyone else.

I have learnt how to listen to them, reassure them, and tell them that I am safe and it is safe to be compassionate with myself. And then I listen instead to another voice. The voice of my heart who tells me I am enough, to stop and rest, and that I've done enough. She tells me to push back gently but firmly on the client and say, sorry, that's not realistic – we have to find a better way to work together and one that's kinder on me.

Journal prompt: Now spend at least 10 minutes journalling about those voices that tell you you're not good enough, or you can't possibly ask for help, or you can't stop. If you feel you would like to, give them names. The clearer you can get about them, the easier they will be to identify when they pop up and – importantly – the more you practise noticing them, the better you become at not allowing them to drive you.

Practice 2: Mirror Work

In this practice you will use a mirror to reflect back to you a different way of relating to yourself. As I have said, perfectionists speak to themselves harshly and judgmentally. They are unkind to themselves and in doing so, they are perpetuating the cycle of feeling unsafe and driving themselves even harder to control their external environment and find some sense of – false – security.

Mirror work comes from the work of Louise Hay, who also wrote a bestselling book, *Mirror Work,* about the subject. It is deep work and the rewards can be profound. As the empowerment coach Natalia Benson says:

It's about getting to know yourself so you can face your life with courage as an aligned and self-aware human being.

Are you ready to try?

I'm offering you two profound exercises. With both of them find a place to do the exercise where you will be undisturbed for 20–30 minutes.

Start by making eye contact with yourself in the mirror. This may feel a bit odd and uncomfortable at first, but stay with it. The key is to witness yourself without judgement. So often, we look at ourselves in the mirror and we judge, criticize, dislike, etc. But, do we really ever simply stand there and see ourselves, without judgement?

Mirror Work Exercise 1: Who Am I?

Sit comfortably facing a mirror. You might like to light a candle before you start and have a journal or notebook close by.

Set aside at least 20 minutes for this exercise.

Gaze into the mirror and say the words out loud 'Who Am I?'

Initially you might 'hear':

- I am a father.
- I am a husband.
- I am a brother.
- I am a friend.
- I am a gym instructor or lawyer or train driver.

I challenge you to keep gazing at the mirror. Take your time. Relax and connect with your breathing and keep going for at least another 5 minutes.

I am a . . .

Miss Trunchbull (your version) might say to you 'What a load of . . . !' or 'This is so boring' or 'What is the point of this ridiculous exercise?'

Notice her and keep going.

Who are you when you get under the layers and roles you play in your life? Who are you *really*?

Who are you really and do you get a chance to be this in your life?

Spend 10 minutes journalling after you have done the mirror inquiry. Have you learnt anything about yourself?

I suggest you repeat this exercise every day for a week or so. Challenge yourself to keep going deeper. Be patient. Get underneath the layers and give yourself a chance to connect with your heart's longing.

Jackie's Story

As Jackie, an intuitive self-care coach, said, 'I remember crying in my early teens when I did this exercise'. She had been conditioned as a child to be strong and grown-up, as her mother had raised her and her siblings single-handedly and, as a psychiatric

(Continued)

nurse, her mother often had to leave them alone at home while she worked hard to support the family. Jackie had had to grow up very quickly to look after herself and her siblings. She always felt the weight of responsibility on her shoulders and while her brothers and sister might leave to go and play with their friends, she felt she had to be the grown-up one and worry until they returned home safely. Often she couldn't sleep at night until her mother was safely home from work and in bed.

Mirror Work Exercise 2: I Love You

This exercise can be surprisingly hard to do. When you are conditioned to speak to yourself harshly, the gentleness of this exercise can be almost overwhelming. Try to stay connected to your breath as you do the exercise and it is lovely to bring some Havening into the exercise whenever you feel the need to.

Sit comfortably facing a mirror. You might like to light a candle before you start and have a journal or notebook close by.

Set aside at least 20 minutes for this exercise.

Gaze into the mirror, look deeply into your eyes, and say the words out loud 'I love you. . . *(your name)*'.

Stay with the exercise for at least 10 minutes.

You may notice resistance to using these words. Miss Trunchbull (your version) might say to you 'How ridiculous', or 'How self-indulgent', or 'Haven't you got something better to be doing?' Notice if she pops up and keep going.

If you can keep going despite the resistance you may notice that emotions arise and it becomes harder for the words to come out. Your voice might drop and your gaze might become softer. Don't forget to hold yourself in a Havening hug if you need to.

If after doing these mirror exercises, you don't feel any different afterwards, don't worry about it. Be patient. Be willing to be vulnerable, and aim to choose one practice at a time and do it at least once a week or, ideally, daily for a week.

These simply practices can be remarkably transformative if you allow them to impact you.

Returning to Jackie's story, she said that, after a while, 'One day the penny dropped that I love myself.' Doing the exercise on a daily basis also brought home to her how unhappy she had been before this.

Practice 3: Let it Out!

Holding in your truth can be exhausting and can cause a myriad of symptoms from teeth grinding to headaches, throat complaints, skin disorders such as eczema, psoriasis, and even acne. But how do you learn how to speak up when you're so used to repressing and holding the words in? How do you learn to express safely?

The following exercise is a great way of releasing the stuck energy of frustration, anger, and the stress from holding in. It is called Lion's Breath or *Simhasana* in Sanskrit. Not only does it help to release pent-up emotions but it can also help with releasing the jaw and alleviating teeth grinding.

You can do Lion's Breath while sitting in a chair or kneeling on all fours. You can also do it sitting cross-legged.

Focus your gaze on the space between your eyebrows or even on the tip of your nose. Or you can open your eyes wide and gaze up toward the ceiling or sky.

1. Lean forward slightly, bracing your hands on your knees or the floor.
2. Spread your fingers as wide as possible.
3. Inhale through your nose.
4. Open your mouth wide, stick out your tongue, and stretch it down toward your chin.
5. Exhale forcefully, carrying the breath across the root of your tongue.
6. While exhaling, make a 'ha' sound that comes from deep within your abdomen.
7. Breathe normally for a few moments.
8. Repeat Lion's Breath up to 7 times.
9. Finish by breathing deeply for 1 to 3 minutes.

Go Deeper

You can go deeper with this practice by setting an intention for your practice. By this I mean, what is it that you really want to say that is frustrating you because you can't say it?

Start your practice by lighting a candle. Then, set an intention to let go of anything you no longer wish to hold on to.

With each exhale, imagine that you are releasing whatever it is that no longer serves you. Notice if you have any resistance to this or are holding on to anything tightly. If this is the case, simply acknowledge it and trust that you can let go when you're ready.

End your practice by thinking about and perhaps journalling about what you would like to call into your life, such as joy, calm, contentment, or peace.

If you have been holding in something you would like to say to someone else but find it hard to, imagine releasing those words into the fire as you perform the exercise. When you are done, close your eyes and peacefully imagine how you would like your relationship with the person to feel now you have expressed your truth.

Many people find that once they have done this exercise, it is so much easier to communicate with this person afterwards. It is really quite magical.

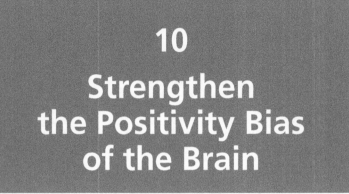

10
Strengthen
the Positivity Bias
of the Brain

'The remedy is not to suppress negative experiences; when they happen, they happen. Rather, it is to foster positive experiences – and in particular, to take them in so they become a permanent part of you.'
—Rick Hanson, *Buddha's Brain: The Practical Neuroscience of Happiness, Love and Wisdom*

How are you feeling right now?

Are you ready to put deep nourishment into your soil? You have 'propped yourself up' with the clean-up, aerated your soul with your breath, and come back to your body. Please can I reassure you that all of this is a work in progress and, as I've said before, the work is never done until we're done, but I'm hoping that by now you are starting to feel more supported, more resourced – and safer.

Let's go deeper . . .

When you are overwhelmed with stress and anxiety, it can be difficult to notice or feel that anything at all is going well in your life. Everything can feel dark and hopeless. This can be made worse by the fact that, for our survival, the brain has evolved with a negativity bias which means it holds on to negative and stressful experiences while not even registering that good ones are also taking place. As the neuroscientist Dr Rick Hanson says: 'The brain is like Velcro for negative experiences and Teflon for positives ones.' His work shows that we can start to grow the positivity bias of the brain by using specific exercises and in so doing, these pathways of the brain are strengthened and can even override old patterns of thinking which no longer serve us.

This isn't about going around in a deluded state of 'toxic positivity'. This isn't about brushing things under the carpet and pretending that our lives are perfect. It especially isn't about invalidating our felt experiences. Rather we are consciously choosing to put our attention and awareness to establishing new neural pathways in the brain that enable us to bypass our default destructive or negative tendencies that are so damaging to our health and innate sense of safety. Martin Seligman, the US psychologist and author of several self-help books, refers to 'realistic optimism' – the ability to balance out the negative and positive in people and situations. It is the ability to explore opportunities and have faith that the future can be better than what has happened in the past.

Many people wake up in a state of fear and anxiety. They fuel it by looking at their phones, disappearing into social media, or watching the news. By then, they have well and truly fallen into a well of despair and worry.

I used to be this way myself and still have mornings when I notice that the old pattern is back. I don't look at my phone but sometimes, for no particular reason, I find myself waking up with my mind filled with old and unhelpful patterns of thinking which, if I allowed them to, could end up running and ruining my day. I could blame this on my upbringing and growing up in a family in which fear and anxiety were the norm. Growing up in Guyana was fraught with risk and for the seven years that I lived there we always had guard dogs and even security guards on our compound. For many years, I had a leaning towards negative thinking and fear – those neural tramlines were well-worn.

Thankfully, we can change and the brain is neuroplastic, which means that new neural pathways can be grown and strengthened, but we do need the right tools and practices and ways of thinking.

One way is by cultivating gratitude. Gratitude for our life, however challenging it might be, gratitude for the people around us and the circumstances we encounter every day from the moment we wake up.

Apparently, the Dalai Lama often says when he wakes up: 'I am fortunate to be alive, I have a precious human life, I am not going to waste it.' He has had a difficult life, being forced to flee his home country of Tibet due to the

Chinese suppression. He now lives in exile in Dharamsala in India and is considered to be a descendent of the Buddha. His teachings are based on gratitude, compassion and kindness, and the philosophy that true happiness and joy come from within and are independent of external circumstances. I also believe this to be true and my work with many people has strengthened this belief; time and again I have seen that it is possible to cultivate a deep sense of wellbeing by paying attention to how we relate to our everyday circumstances. How this relates to feeling safe is that when we go through life seeing everything as a threat, we become activated and triggered, our nervous system in hyper-alert sympathetic mode. On the other hand, the more we attune ourselves to noticing the good, even small glimpses of good, the more this calms our nervous system so we live more from our safety ventral vagus mode.

The beauty of this work lies in the fact that we can retrain our brains to start to notice the good, so not only does our environment start to feel less hostile but we stop living in fear and anticipating threat.

I am going to share with you some exercises based on gratitude and appreciation. They are simple but they work powerfully to thaw out trapped emotions and to bring more lightness to your heart. For years I have been recommending these practices to clients with sleep problems and realized that it was having an incredible effect on their ability not only to sleep well but to face their life problems with courage and resilience. In other words, they were feeling safer to do life! I share them with you with an open heart and pray that they can make a difference for you too.

Practice 1: Gratitude for the Present Moment

It is good to do this practice as a meditation or a journalling exercise.

Sit comfortably in a chair with your back supported and your feet firmly planted on the ground. You can also do this sitting cross-legged if that is comfortable for you.

Take a deep breath in through your nose and out through your mouth. Do this again and allow yourself to relax into the moment, feeling the relaxation in your body and holding awareness of the areas of your body that are touching the chair or the ground.

Now I'd like you to reflect on this question: Who or what are you feeling grateful for *right now* in this present moment?

If you are new to this sort of exercise, you might not be able to bring anything to mind and you may need to dig a bit deeper. Has anything happened in your day so far that you are grateful for? Has anything happened that feels good – even a nice shower or a perfect cup of tea? Has anyone said anything nice to you or sent you a nice text message?

What has happened in your day so far that you can feel grateful for in this moment?

Take some time to bring the memory to life. Relive and soak in the positive experience. Remember the person's face or how the words made you feel. Whatever it is that you are grateful for, spend some time – even a minute – remembering and enjoying the experience.

As you do this, say out loud or silently 'thank you'. If you've remembered many things (well done!) say 'thank you' as you take your time and light your attention on each positive thing, no matter how small.

As you go about your day, I challenge you to notice every time something good happens and to say thank you, out loud or in your mind.

Let this be your thank you prayer. Cultivate gratitude as you go about your day.

When you say thank you, who are you thanking? This depends on your beliefs. Maybe a higher power or angels. You might be thanking God or Allah or maybe yourself for making these positive things happen.

Whatever your belief, gratitude is a powerful way of strengthening neural connections in the brain that create inner safety and calm in the body.

Practice 2: Wake up with Gratitude

When you wake up, even before you have opened your eyes and especially before you have looked at your phone, simply say 'thank you'.

Even if you haven't slept particularly well, say thank you for the rest that you have had, the comfortable bed you sleep in, the safe space of your room, the opportunity to rest for a minute or so right now before you move into your day.

Start your day with gratitude.

Practice 3: End Your Day with Gratitude

When you turn your light out, settle down into your bed and as your eyes close, say 'thank you' for the day you have had. Go backwards through your day, place your attention on every small positive thing that happened in your day and say thank you silently. If you wake during the night, say thank you for this time to rest or you can even go backwards through your day again and give thanks – it is a powerful way of falling asleep again.

You can also do this exercise as a journalling practice to end your day.

Practice 4: Cultivate Appreciation

This is another simple but profound way of bringing feelings of safety into your body as you go about your busy day. It is particularly helpful to use this practice if you're feeling anxious or worried.

The practice is to simply notice and appreciate the small occurrences in your day as they happen. For example, if you're going for a walk set your intention before you step out of the front door to appreciate anything good – however small, you come across in your walk:

- Thank you for this sunshine on my face.
- Thank you for the warmth of this jacket I am wearing.
- Thank you for that person who smiled at me.
- Thank you for this feeling of walking and breathing in fresh air.
- Thank you that even though it is raining and I'm getting wet I am not cold.
- Thank you for the vitality I feel in my body as I walk.
- Thank you for the feeling of my feet on the ground as I walk.
- Thank you for this time to take a walk.

Do you see how easy it is? This exercise also brings you into the present moment and can be particularly helpful if you are feeling fearful or anxious. You become aware of what is happening right here and right now in your body, noticing your surroundings instead of getting caught up in swirling, anxiety-laden thoughts.

Sometimes when people start using these practices they feel a bit stuck. As Sarah said when she first started: 'Nothing good has happened in my day so far'. Then, I gently guided her to remember that her boyfriend had given her a lovely hug before he left for work, that she'd had a relaxing warm bath, and that she'd had a nice chat with her mother in the morning.

Our survival instinct and negatively biased brains always want us to look for what is wrong. We are not primed to look for what is right and there is always something to be grateful for, even on our darkest days. Your challenge is to start looking deeper, to start noticing, to start acknowledging that the good is there if you are prepared to see and feel it.

Practice 5: Soak in Pleasure

When you do something that makes you feel good – listening to music, dancing, soaking in a hot bath, etc., really allow yourself to sink into the feeling of pleasure. Savour it. Allow it to linger with you. Breathe into it. Allow the feelings to soften you. Lying in bed first thing in the morning or last thing at night – allow yourself to soak up the pleasure of the sensations, let them seep into your cells. Breathe them in deeply. Say to yourself 'this feels so good'.

The use of the word 'soak' is deliberate. Remember, the brain tends to have a negativity bias so we really need to tell it that something good is happening and let it 'marinate' in the experience. Taking the time to do this is what starts to create stronger neural connections of positivity and hope. Tell your brain that you are receiving pleasure, tell it a bit more and then a bit more and it will start to become more and more receptive to it.

There are a myriad of small ways in which we can begin to cultivate pleasure. The more we practise doing it, the better we get at generating inner joy rather than constantly looking outside of ourselves for external stimuli to make us feel good. For example:

- After your bath or shower, take time to anoint your body with lotion or oil and enjoy the sensation of doing this.
- Savour your cup of tea as you drink it. Really take your time over it rather than gulping it down. Enjoy the warmth from the cup and the flavour of the tea.
- Stroke your pet and enjoy the sensation of their soft silky fur and their pleasure at being stroked. Notice how they bask in your attention.
- Enjoy the feeling of being able to rest in a comfy chair after a hard day of work.

- Enjoy silence – this is one that I particularly enjoy but for some people it might take a bit of working at. When you come home or while driving in the car, avoid putting the television or radio on. Bask in the silence for a little while, allow yourself to feel calm and peace descending as you learn to appreciate quiet.

Practice 6: Morning Intention Setting

When you wake up in the morning,
leave your phone untouched.
Keep your energy with you, rather than projected into your day, already.
Keep your eyes closed. Simply meet yourself.
Be with whatever is there.
Be with you before you be with them.
Maybe you will encounter fear, worry, sadness.
But maybe you will find joy and glee for your day.
Who knows? Every day is different.
Get to know who you are.
Learn to listen to the longings of your soul.
They will guide you.
Get to know your breath and where it wants to go.
Where the soil has become compacted and wants more.
Allow yourself to uncover your yearnings.
Who knows what you will find?
Embrace your fears and ...
Show you who you are.
Know who you are.
Be who you are.
You are safe.

11
Safety in Connection

'The pandemic has shown us that people need relationships.'
—Sherry Turkle, author of *Alone Together*

Earlier in my book, I described the importance of 'social engagement' and how important it is that we connect with others in meaningful and nourishing ways. Over the years, many people have become starved of meaningful connection as cursory interactions on social media have become the way to connect. However, an unexpected and positive side effect of the Covid-19 pandemic after months of social distancing and social isolation was that many people realized how much they needed other people and true relating. They realized how much they needed to see other people smile genuine smiles that reached their eyes, to hug and feel the touch of another human being. Loneliness was one of the biggest 'illnesses' during this time and many people reported feeling depressed and even suicidal.

Making New Friends

I lived in this neighbourhood for five years before the pandemic hit and while I was always happy to smile and make passing small talk about the weather to my neighbours, I'd never really formed deep connections with any of them. In March 2020, when the first lockdown hit the UK, I started going down to the river to swim most days. Invariably, people would come and talk to me. When I got my dog, my community grew even more and now, it's unusual for me to step outside of my house and not have someone to talk to. Years ago, as a bit of an introvert, I might have thought this tiresome but now I revel in the smiles and chats with my neighbours and the people I meet on my dog walks and by the river. I sometimes leave my house feeling a little lonely or sad and return feeling nourished and filled up with good interactions. I now have 'river friends' who I know will be friends for a very long time.

When we are trusting, compassionate, and warm-hearted, we attract exactly that back into our lives. We create an atmosphere around us that is positive and friendly. We see friends everywhere. If you go around in a state of fear and distrust, people feel it and they distance themselves. Then we start to feel unlovable and lonely. If you walk around judging others, you exude

this energy and will appear unapproachable to other
people. Often this is a defence mechanism against hurt
and rejection so we tell ourselves:

I don't get him.
He doesn't get me.
They're not on my wavelength.
I just don't fit in.
I'm better than them.
They think they're better than me.

What if loneliness is an illusion that we have got caught
up in? We all have days when we feel lonely, but the very
idea of loneliness comes from the false notion that we
are separate and isolated parts in a world filled with
other separate, isolated parts. Human beings are social
animals; we are all connected and we can all start to
experience a deep sense of belonging, rootedness, and
safety if we allow ourselves to tap into this interconnectedness. How do we do this?

Yet again, we can learn from nature and trees. Scientists –
notably Peter Wohlleben – have discovered that trees
talk to each other via networks of fine hairs growing
from root tips which join with microscopic fungal fila-
ments to form the basic links of a communication network between trees. These networks are called
mycorrhizal networks and they enable trees – and even
trees of different species – to 'speak' to each other. The
scientists even refer to this network as the 'wood wide

web'. In other words, trees reach out to each other. They thrive through their interconnection – as can we.

All of nature is interconnected. We are all connected. When we start to realize this and feel this, our loneliness begins to melt away. We start to experience deep belonging.

But how do we cultivate connection in these lonely 'world wide web' times? First of all, we have to be receptive to trusting others and opening our hearts and minds to connecting with other people and even strangers. This doesn't usually happen overnight especially if we've been conditioned by our past life experiences not to trust others. Or we might have told ourselves we don't need other people, that we're best off going it alone. Bear in mind, feelings of self-sufficiency that stem from distrust and lack of safety could go way back into your ancestry – these feelings and patterns might not even belong to you! The fact is that even though hell can sometimes be other people, research strongly indicates that loneliness and social isolation are a major source of mental illness and unhappiness. Today's world can be so divisive – you and me, them and us. It is time to recognize and find safety in our common humanity. Time to remind ourselves that despite appearances and fear of rejection, we really are deeply connected even though we can't see it.

Here are some profound practices that I have adapted from Deb Dana's work along with Buddhist practices and some of the powerful practices I've personally discovered along the way.

Practice 1: Prepare Your Heart Connection

I believe this to be an invaluable exercise to do if you have decided that you really do want to connect with other people, to open yourself to trusting others and inviting in new friendships. Or maybe you want to connect more deeply with your existing friends or family members.

This beautiful practice works on the basis of activating the Social Engagement System that resides at the base of your skull.

Before you start, hold in your mind the intention to connect more openly and deeply with others.

Now place your hands at the base of your skull. Allow the weight of your head to rest in your hands. Rest here for a minute or so with eyes open or closed.

Move your hands so one hand rests on the side of your face and the other rests over your heart. Breathe into this posture and imagine the energy flowing between your face and your heart. See it like a circuit of energy flowing from face to heart and back in the other direction between heart and face. Allow yourself to soften into the flow of energy. Feel your eyes and face soften and relax. This heart-face connection is a vital part of our social engagement system and when we activate it in this way, we create around us an aura of friendliness and approachability. It is also an effective way of soothing our own feelings of lack of confidence and safety to interact with others.

Breathe deeply in this posture for a minute or two and as you do so imagine roots growing from your feet grounding you and connecting you to all of life. Imagine sending your positive intention to connect out into the world.

Practice 2: Meditation for Loneliness

This exercise is based on a beautiful Buddhist practice. Regardless of your beliefs, we can all benefit from doing it. It becomes even more powerful if you do the previous practice before this one.

Step 1 – Imagine someone you love – a child, a parent, a close friend, or a cherished pet. Bring their image into your mind and allow yourself to feel the love you have for them. You can use the heart-face posture described in Practice 1 while doing this. Notice feelings of warmth, softness, and openheartedness that spread through your body as you allow the feelings of love for them.

Step 2 – Now imagine someone you know but do not know well – this might be a colleague at work or a neighbour, or someone who works in your local supermarket.

Recognize how different your feelings are for this person compared to the person you just had in mind. How do you feel about them? You might feel a small amount of warmth or empathy. On the other hand, you might feel indifferent. Can you imagine their life, their desire for happiness, their hopes and dreams, their suffering? Can you feel a sense of connection with their experience and common humanity? They might also experience loneliness – just as you do – and when you connect with them in this way, your reaching out strengthens the web of interconnection.

Step 3 – Take this awareness and receptivity into the world as you go about your day. You do not have to wait for others to open their hearts to you before you open yours. By opening yours and being more receptive, you will notice that you feel more connected to others wherever you go.

Before you leave your home to go for a walk or a trip to the supermarket, set an intention to smile at other people. Don't take your phone with you. Go on your walk with an inner smile. Experiment with softening your gaze and making gentle eye contact with others if it feels right to – the more you practise doing this, the easier it becomes to gauge whether it is actually safe to smile or talk with a stranger. Talk to the staff at your local supermarket, get to know their names. I now know that at my local supermarket Hazel loves gardening, Bubaka is studying for a degree in computer science, and Anton is trying to give up smoking.

Put your phone away and practise connecting with others. Enjoy developing feelings of empathy and compassion for people you don't know. Enjoy the feelings of belonging and connection that this brings you.

Practice 3: Deep Support

We all need support in life. We may feel we need to go our own way, that we can't reach out to others, but the reality is that we're not meant to exist in isolation – an important aspect of thriving is knowing when to lean up against friends, family, or professional help.

Friendship can come in many forms and it can fulfil many different needs. We might have friends who we can laugh with, who we can share a glass of wine with. They might also be friends who we can rant or cry with. We might have friends who are fun but we don't go so deep with them.

This is a reflection exercise that is best done by journalling.

- Who or what is supporting you *deeply* in your life?
- Who can you laugh with?
- Who can you cry with?

Spend at least a few minutes reflecting and writing about these questions.

Your support may also come from non-human sources – for example, my dog is one of my biggest supports, as is walking in nature or swimming in the river.

What resources are available in your life right now?

If doing this exercise has made you aware that you really don't have enough support around you, how can you increase your level of support?

Sarah's Story

When I asked Sarah to think about the support in her life, she became quite emotional when she realized that she was used to assuming the role of carer and confidante. Usually her friends came to her with their problems and worries. She was the one who often provided a shoulder to cry on, but it wasn't reciprocated. I asked her if she ever asked for support from her friends and family and she realized that she didn't. We discussed whether she felt safe enough to express herself honestly in these relationships and she said she didn't because she was afraid of being judged. She was in a very thoughtful mood when we ended the session.

A few weeks later I saw Sarah for a catch-up and she was visibly brighter. She was going to a comedy

(Continued)

show with her friend who felt Sarah needed cheering up and had started talking more openly and freely with her mother and brother. She was surprised at how receptive and caring they had been.

Creating deep support for ourselves requires an openness to sharing and being vulnerable. It requires trust in both ourselves and others.

I invite you to repeat the following affirmation every morning as soon as you wake up and, as always, before you open your eyes. Take a few deep breaths before starting to create a state of receptivity and say:

- I am open to receive the support and love of those people around me.
- I am open to receive the abundant support of the Universe around me . . . and I am looking forward to receiving it.

Repeat this affirmation every morning for at least one week.

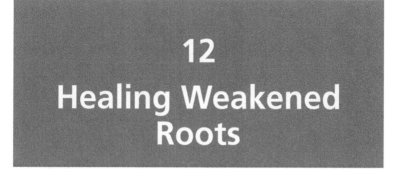

12
Healing Weakened Roots

'Traumas do not sleep, even with death, but rather continue to look for the fertile ground of resolution in the children of the following generations.'
—Norman Doidge, MD., *The Brain That Changes Itself: Stories of Personal Triumph From the Frontiers of Brain Science*

Earlier I shared the story of my family lineage in the hope that it would inspire you to think about your own roots and where you have come from. At the time of writing this book, I continue to do the work on my ancestral trauma and the weakened roots of my family lineage. My journey, *the* journey, is ongoing. But as each layer of healing takes place I settle more deeply into my life and into my body. I feel safer and I sleep more deeply.

Practice 1: Explore Your Family Tree

I now offer you some gentle reflective questions to set you on your way to beginning an investigation into your family history. You may choose to reflect on these questions as simple meditation or journalling exercises or alongside working with a trained therapist. These are questions that invite you to go deep. You might just choose to reflect on one of them for a few days. Take your time, don't feel you have to rush them:

- Who are you and where do you come from?
- Have you ever explored the stories of your ancestors?
- Do any stories particularly stand out in your mind and if so, why?
- Do you have a relative or grandparent with whom you have a particular affinity (even if you never met them in person)?
- When do you feel this connection with them?
- What do they represent for you?
- Can you start to unpick the roots that have made you who you are and see how they have got you to where you are now?
- Can you see how they connect with your personality and the traits you express now?
- Can you see which ones have stood you in good stead and where they came from?
- Can you identify the roots that need some healing?
- There may be areas in life where your growth is stunted or you hold back, feeling limited in some way.
- What are the roots that need nourishing?
- Where do you feel held back, limited from thriving and achieving your full potential?

Write down your answers and reflect on them for several days – don't expect instant answers. Let them work their magic on your understanding and gain the maximum benefit from answering these questions from an open heart. In so doing you give yourself a great chance to bring about your healing as well as that of your family line, and to ensure your own feeling of being safe, right now.

You can explore your family dynamic further in **family constellation circles**. This considers an individual as part of a larger constellation of their family members, even ancestors from many generations before, meaning that their behaviours, feelings, and attitudes must be understood within this context. Every family operates with its own unspoken rules, and family constellation circles can uncover hidden dynamics and entanglements that are repeated across generations.

Practice 2: Tree Meditation Exercise

I want to share with you a meditation that I practise very often as well as recommending it to many clients. I have my favourite trees that I go to near my home beside the River Thames but sometimes I simply close my eyes and use my imagination.

This meditation is a pretty simple one and is best practised without anything to distract you (notably your mobile phone). I recommend that you read through the exercise a few times and then simply do it without any prompts. There's no right or wrong way of doing it and you can make it your own. Enjoy it and notice the benefits you feel as you go about the rest of your day.

I invite you, when you are next out walking in nature, to pay close attention to the trees around you.

Are you drawn to a particular tree? If not, find a tree that appeals to you and stand at its foot. It would be good if you could take your shoes off and sit under the tree. But you don't have to, simply standing by the tree is enough. As you gaze at the tree, keep your awareness on your feet. Feel them firmly planted on the ground.

Can you see the roots of the tree? If not, can you imagine the root plate of the tree lying beneath the soil, strongly anchoring this tree into the ground, keeping it safe?

Now take a deep breath in and send your out breath down and out through your feet. Imagine you are breathing out thick roots from the soles of your feet. Imagine those roots growing down and through the soil and meeting and merging with the roots of the tree. Feel yourself becoming more anchored to the earth, grounded, steady, and safe.

Feel the connection between yourself and this tree. Feel the tree protecting you, keeping you rooted and safe. If you are feeling any fears or anxieties, imagine breathing them out of you and sending them down through your tree roots and into the soil. Breathe them out.

Allow this tree to show you how to find safety in your body, how to be safe. You can come back to her anytime and even in your imagination, simply close your eyes and imagine yourself in front of your special tree taking comfort, protection, and strength from her. Allowing her to remind you that you really are safe . . . all you need to do is come back to yourself, come back to your body, feel your feet and breathe.

Epilogue: Return Home

'We are not human beings having a spiritual experience.
We are spiritual beings having a human experience.'
—Pierre Teilhard de Chardin

Ultimately, the journey to feeling safe is a journey of coming home. Coming back home to the body, our safe container. Coming back to ourselves and our souls.

In the process of keeping up with life, we've lost our way. We've forgotten why we're really here.

We look outside of ourselves to keep safe, seeking control of our external environment and often tying ourselves up into tightly wound perfectionistic knots in the process.

Maybe we – our lives – need to unravel before we can find true safety.

Maybe we need to face our worst fears before we can find true safety.

Yes, this work – the Real Work – takes courage. Returning home to the body is like coming home when you have been gone for a long time. You could find rooms and corners that are dark and dusty because they were locked and abandoned for so long. Coming back can be scary. During the pandemic, so many people had strange dreams. I was interviewed many times for TV and radio about these 'lockdown dreams' that so many people were experiencing. The most common one was about discovering hidden rooms, attics, and cellars that you didn't know were in your home. People were having these dreams because they had been forced throughout lockdown to be introspective, to open those inner doors and face their demons. Many discovered new aspects to themselves, finding new levels of trust and faith – they found inner safety.

You have to be brave to open those doors. But the rewards are so great when you start to tap into a well-spring of hope, faith, trust, joy – all of the things that make us feel safe. Not only do you feel it, but you start to exude it like a fire glow to those around you – your children, the people you love, your friends, your colleagues, the world around you. Don't we all want to live in a world that feels safer? Of course we do and so we have to become the change that we want to see in the world. To do this we have to remember who we are and who we aren't.

In the last year, while writing this book I suffered a devastating and totally unexpected personal loss. I found myself in a deep dark place that I hadn't been in for decades and had thought I would never return to again. But evidently not. I was back in this place and I wasn't even sure if I had the energy to leave it. Eventually, I began to see glimmers and glimpses of light and so I began my journey back. This time was different though. This time I had even more resources, a bulging toolkit and a deep sense of faith that everything would be all right in the end.

And it is. Today, as I sit and write these words, I marvel at how far I've come in the last months. I marvel at the cracks and crevices I've found myself going into so I can sit here and write from my truth because I believe that the writing of *Finding Inner Safety* has had to come from some considerable depths, from some unearthing. This book has been in the writing for more than 15 years and it comes from my soul. I've shown up at the keyboard – at times when I haven't wanted to – and I've written, and what has emerged for me is a sense of peace, contentment, and inner safety such as I have never known. I feel I am truly and unashamedly thriving!

I want this for you and I want it for our world too. There is too much fear around us and in the last year, even more so. People are afraid to leave their homes, to hug, to even smile at strangers. I believe people are even afraid to thrive. Everywhere I go people say 'I'm surviving' as if it is not possible to thrive in these times – and it's not surprising when, all around us, the messages are strong and negative – the world is not safe. Maybe this is true on some levels. Our world will always be fraught with fear and things to be afraid of. But what I know is that we can choose to navigate this world of un-safety from a place of safety that resides within us – within all of us – and in so doing, we give ourselves a chance to thrive. We are physiologically designed for both un-safety and for safety. Every day and in every moment we can make a choice about where we want to live from. But we each have to make that choice.

The Salt Path by Raynor Winn tells the true story of a husband and wife in their fifties who, by sheer bad luck, lost their home and everything they owned to debt collectors. As if things really couldn't get worse, the husband was diagnosed with a crippling terminal illness. With literally only pennies in their pocket, they decide to walk the UK's 630-mile South West Coast path. Things go from bad to worse when the husband runs out of his pain medication and goes into withdrawal. But as the story unravels, living wild and free, surrounded by nature, they find inner safety and peace.

In her memoir *Dying to Be Me*, Anita Moorjani describes how after her extraordinary near-death experience (NDE) she discovered the true purpose of her life. She didn't realize this until her NDE. Her story is remarkable; she was diagnosed with stage IV cancer and was lying in intensive care dying. To all intents and purposes, she *did* die – but she chose to come back. In doing so, her life changed, she changed. She has now become a leading spiritual teacher and guide who urges us to make the most of our lives while we're here and to not forget our true nature – our spiritual nature.

But so many of us do.

In my work I have had the immense privilege to watch countless other people embark on similar journeys. As well, I have watched many others become dispirited and burnt out, as they continue to look outside of themselves to feel safe. Many of the corporate environments in which I consult are tough places for people to work. They are paid well but at what cost? Not surprisingly, these are the environments that seem to have the highest rates of burnout and people don't feel safe. To me, they feel soulless. Not surprising that so many people become dispirited.

My work is about connecting people with their spirit. It is my *dharma*, my soul purpose. It's about reminding them what is the greatest source of their energy, the ultimate way of resting peacefully, the best route to truly feeling safe and experiencing a joyful life. Now, more than ever, we need to remember. The price of forgetting is too high. We suffer, our children suffer, and generations to come will suffer. Let us choose differently, let us choose to remember.

What are we choosing to remember? In Zen Buddhism there is a saying 'Show me your original face before you were born'. A variation is 'Without thinking of good or evil, show me your original face before your mother and father were born'. This asks us to stretch back in time to our real and authentic self – the self we are and were before we were born. But how do we remember and experience this right now, in our everyday lives when we're feeling afraid, confused, so busy that we feel perpetually chased? Stop, pause right now and allow yourself to be with this present moment – as I've shown you many times in this book. Breathe deeply, feel your feet on the ground. Do this many times – there is always time – there are 1440 minutes in a day, after all. I promise you, if you do this enough times you will discover something within you. Something that guides you. That protects you and holds you safe even while all around you things are swirling and chaotic.

Right now, before you put this book down, relax for a moment and take a deep breath, place your hand over your heart, and ask yourself – now you have read my book – what one step you can take right now that will contribute the most to your finding deep inner safety. Then take it!

About the Author

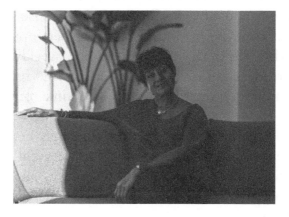

Dr Nerina Ramlakhan has worked as a physiologist and sleep expert for 25 years. She spent a decade conducting sleep and wellness programmes at the Capio Nightingale Hospital in London, coaches on burnout prevention at Ashridge Business School, and is the original founder of BUPA's Corporate Wellbeing Solutions. Nerina works with individuals as well as numerous corporate clients from various industries including sport (Chelsea Football Club) and hosts a regular sleep programme at Vale de Moses yoga retreat, Portugal.

Nerina is the author of *Tired But Wired* (Souvenir Press, 2010); *Fast Asleep, Wide Awake* (Thorsons, 2016); and *The Little Book of Sleep: The Art of Natural Sleep* (Gaia, 2018). Her work has been featured in *The Times, The Telegraph, The Guardian, New Scientist, Psychologies, Red,* and *Healthy Living* magazines and she has appeared on numerous national TV and radio programmes including *This Morning, Jamie and Jimmy's Friday Night Feast, Sky News,* and BBC Radio 2. Nerina is also a *Stylist* editorial contributor and gives her expert opinion for the Stylist Sleep Diaries, an ongoing weekly feature where readers can record their routines and receive her expert advice on their lifestyle and bedtime routines.

As a former insomniac, Nerina combines her professional experience with academic and personal insights, and believes sleep problems are not simply about sleep, but rather about how we deal with life and its inevitable challenges.

Nerina enjoys yoga, meditation, and climbing. She used to enjoy running and cycling and completed seven marathons and several triathlons. She's now an avid wild swimmer and is often to be found in the Thames while being watched over by her faithful pup, Mira. She has a seventeen-year-old daughter and lives in London.